Mnemonics in

HOSPITAL MANAGEMENT

Mnemonics in HOSPITAL MANAGEMENT

HB Parmar
MBA (Hospital Management) PGDHHM BHMS DNHE
Public Health Manager
Department of Health
Corporation Program Management Unit
Rajkot Municipal Corporation
Rajkot, Gujarat, India

Foreword
Vijay Pandya

JAYPEE *The Health Sciences Publisher*
New Delhi | London | Panama

JAYPEE Jaypee Brothers Medical Publishers (P) Ltd.

Headquarters
Jaypee Brothers Medical Publishers (P) Ltd.
4838/24, Ansari Road, Daryaganj
New Delhi 110 002, India
Phone: +91-11-43574357
Fax: +91-11-43574314
E-mail: jaypee@jaypeebrothers.com

Overseas Offices

J.P. Medical Ltd.
83, Victoria Street, London
SW1H 0HW (UK)
Phone: +44- 20 3170 8910
Fax: +44(0) 20 3008 6180
E-mail: info@jpmedpub.com

Jaypee Highlights Medical Publishers Inc.
City of Knowledge, Building 235, 2nd Floor
Clayton, Panama City, Panama
Phone: +1 507-301-0496
Fax: +1 507-301-0499
E-mail: cservice@jphmedical.com

Jaypee Brothers Medical Publishers (P) Ltd.
17/1-B, Babar Road, Block-B, Shaymali
Mohammadpur, Dhaka-1207
Bangladesh
Mobile: +08801912003485
E-mail: jaypeedhaka@gmail.com

Jaypee Brothers Medical Publishers (P) Ltd.
Bhotahity, Kathmandu, Nepal
Phone: +977-9741283608
E-mail: kathmandu@jaypeebrothers.com

Website: www.jaypeebrothers.com
Website: www.jaypeedigital.com

Inquiries for bulk sales may be solicited at: jaypee@jaypeebrothers.com

Mnemonics in Hospital Management

First Edition: **2017**

ISBN: 978-93-5270-096-7

Printed at Rajkamal Electric Press, Plot No. 2, Phase-IV, Kundli, Haryana.

Dedicated to

My honorable teacher and management guru

Dr Sharad Vyas

His inspiration and encouragement precipitates me to write this book

Foreword

It is my proud privilege to write the foreword for *Mnemonics in Hospital Management* by Dr HB Parmar. Public Health Manager, Dr HB Parmar, an eminent scholar from Rajkot, Gujarat, India, is well versed with the need of healthcare professionals and has expertise in writing such books.

In this creative book, various topics of healthcare management are narrated in an easy-to-memorize method, so that anybody can recall the subject matter very easily. The author has written the book for the perspective of professional people in a lucid manner with some emphasises on administrator's appeal, keywords explanation, health legislation, quotations on health, management explanation, and last but not least valuable tips on management mantra.

Nowadays, many books are available on healthcare and hospital management but this unique book will be equally useful to the students as well as administrators and professional doctors who have very busy schedule in their practice and day-to-day managerial issues of the hospital.

I wish him success in his endeavor and glad to release this innovative book.

Vijay Pandya
MBBS MD (Community Medicine) PGDHHM
Chief Health Officer (Class I)
Rajkot Municipal Corporation
Dr Ambedkar Bhavan
Rajkot, Gujarat, India

Preface

The word mnemonic is derived from the ancient Greek word *Mnemonikos* (*of memory*) and is related to *Mnemosyne* (*remembrance*), the name of the Goddess of memory in Greek mythology. Both of these terms refer back to Mnema (*remembrance*). Mnemonics in antiquity were most considered in the context of what is recently known as an Art of Memory.

Mnemonics is based on associations with easy-to-remember constructs which can be related back to the data that is to be remembered. This is based on the principle that the human mind much more easily remembers spatial, personal, surprising, humorous or otherwise meaningful information than arbitrary sequences. Mnemonics come in many varieties, and can aid memorization of many types of information easily. Where there is something to remember, mnemonics can be put to use.

Mnemonic is a pattern of words used to aid the memory and learning process. It is a special method to improve the memory. Mnemonic device dramatically improves the memory. Sometimes, we use many words without knowing its full form, such as LASER, an acronym and short form of Light Amplification by Stimulated Emission of Radiation. Instead of this long phrase, LASER can be easily recalled and remembered. Mnemonic devices are strategies to improve memory by organizing information. This style of presentation often stimulates the memory.

Nowadays, hospital management is coming up as a distinct specialty. Subject is very vast; issues and information are enormous, as it is merging of two broad specialties—medicine and management. There is pouring of data in this field day-by-day. This unique book contains information on various topics of health and hospital management in a special style. It is not an easy task to present all the topics into mnemonic form, still there is potent scope in this direction. For easy reference, an exhaustive list of contents is presented in beginning of the book. A book of this nature calls for gleaning upon the subject matter from reliable sources, and presenting it in an easily memorizing method. The treatment of the topic is lucid and its coverage is comprehensive. The book contains more than

200 topics in mnemonic form, many meanings of management, and last but not least keywords explanation. The book is equally useful to students, doctors, professionals and all, who are concerned with health and hospital management.

I would like to thank to all my honorable teachers, colleagues, critics, friends, family members, well-wishers and all, who have nourished this work, but my special thanks to M/s Jaypee Brothers Medical Publishers (P) Ltd, New Delhi, India, who have given helping hand by publishing this book. Any suggestions for the improvement of the book would be welcomed, gratefully acknowledged, and used in the subsequent edition.

HB Parmar

Contents

Mnemonics

1. HUMAN RELATIONS

(*Mnemonic:* Human Relations)

H Honest and have self-confidence
U Understand human behavior
Understand other's point of view
M Make yourself a friend of all
A Admit it when you are wrong
N Never make promises which cannot be kept
R Respect and courtesy are important
E Explain thoroughly
L Look, listen and learn all the time (3L)
A Avoid arguments
T Try to be approachable
I Insist on selfless service
O Others first, self second
N Never criticize in public
S Stress the positive always, sociable.

- Human relations refer to the interaction of people in all walks of life.
- It is an art of getting along with people either as individuals or as a group.
- It is the study of the practical attempts to achieve the two separate goals of—greater productivity at work and greater human satisfaction with an organization.
- The basic themes in human relation are related to communication, motivation, responsibility and empathy.

2. PRIMARY HEALTH CARE

Components of Primary Health Care/Elements of Essential Health Care

(*Mnemonic:* ENDEMICS)

E Education to people regarding health
N Nutritional aspect
D Drug supply (rational and essential)
E *Endemic disease:* Prevention and control
M Maternal and child health and family planning services

I Immunization against infectious diseases
C *Common disease and injury:* Proper treatment
S Safe water supply and sanitation.

(These are eight essential elements of Primary Health Care (PHC) as described by the WHO. The concept of PHC has been accepted by all countries. It has also been accepted as an integral part of healthcare delivery system in the country.)

3. TOTAL QUALITY MANAGEMENT

Factors to be Considered are:
(*Mnemonic:* TQM PRINCIPLE)

T Top management leadership
Q Quality management and statistical reports
M Marking of benches
P Process focus
R Recognition and reward
I Improve quality by creation of organizational framework
N Novel approach introduce within health sector
C Customer centered
I Integration of management
P Percolation of hospital work culture
L Learn by practice and teaching
E Employees education and training.

[Total quality management (TQM) is one of the most promising managerial innovations introduced within the health sector. It increases the efficiency and effectiveness of healthcare services. When people are managed according to TQM principles, everyone is more likely to get the employment opportunities and high quality goods and services they demand.]

4. COST ANALYSIS

Pre-requisites of Cost Analysis
(*Mnemonic:* COST)

C Cost center identification
O Organization chart and a chart of accounts relating to it

S System for accurate accounting and comprehensive information
T Tools and techniques for cost analysis.

(Cost analysis is the process of rearranging the data in the existing account to obtain the cost of services rendered by the hospital.
Direct Accounting Approach and Statistical Approach are two general approaches of cost analysis in health sector. For financial management in hospital, process of cost analysis has become a resources tool.)

5. BUDGET

Functional Classification of Budget
(*Mnemonic:* SPONCERS)

S Sale budget
P Planned budget
O Operational budget
N Nonplanned budget
C Cash budget
E Expenditure budget
R Revenue budget
S Summary budget (Master budget).

(Budget is a statement of plans expressed in quantitative, usually in financial term, covering specific period of time, usually one year. It is an important tool for financial planning and control, helps in efficiency, education and expenditures. It is prepared in advanced, derived from long-term strategies and focuses on future.)

6. HOSPITAL ACQUIRED INFECTION

Hospital Acquired Infection: Prevention and Control
(*Mnemonic:* CLEAN WASH)

C CSSD, CHIEF (Chemical, Heat, Ionizing, Ethylene oxide, Filtration)
L Linen and laundry
E Engineering service department
A Antibiotic policy
N Nursing service (Aseptic nursing care can reduce hospital acquired infection)

W Waste management, water supply
A Air conditioning, At cafeteria
S Security (Restricting visitors with security services reduces HAI)
H House-keeping should be efficient.

(HAI also known as Nosocomial Infection and can be defined as "infection acquired by the person in the hospital, manifestation may occur during hospitalization or after discharge from the hospital".
The person may be a patient, hospital staff and/or visitors.
HAI remains a problem all over the world.
According to WHO survey, the prevalence rate of HAI of different hospitals varies from 3–21% with mean of 8.4%.
Litigation on account of HAI due to hospital authority negligence including doctors can be potential litigation under CPA.
HAI attributes large amount of morbidity and mortality and loss of scarce hospital resources. It is in the interest of all of us that HAI will be eradicated!)

7. DIMENSION OF MANAGERIAL INCOMPETENCE

(*Mnemonic:* I AM LEADER)

I *Imaginative:* Impulsive decision, bad ideas
A Arrogant (Narcissistic feelings of entitlement)
M Mistrustful and vindictive
Manages by crises (Colorful)
Mischievous: Careless about commitments, constant lying (Politicians)
L *Leisurely:* Passive-aggressive meanness
Lack of decision (Cautious)
E *Excitable:* Erratic emotional outbursts
A All time Warner
D *Diligent:* Over-controlling micro-manager
Dutiful: Too concerned about pleasing superiors
E Erratic emotional outbursts
R Risk averse (Cautious)

8. DIMENSION OF PERFORMANCE

(Dimensions of Accreditation)

Factors Affecting Patient's Satisfaction (In Terms of Quality of Care)

(*Mnemonic:* A SECRET)

A Availability, Appropriateness
S Safety
E Effectiveness
C Caring and continuity
R Respect
E Efficiency and Efficacy
T Timeliness.

(In the absence of the above-mentioned factors, patient could feel ignored and uncared for their course of the hospital stay.)

9. DISABILITIES

Causes of Disabilities

(*Mnemonic:* MEDICAL CAUSES OF DISABILITIES)

M Malformation of gut and gastrointestinal tract (GIT)
Mental retardation, Malnutrition, Meningitis
E Exposure to toxic substances
D Drug abuse
I Injuries
C Coronary heart disease, Communicable diseases
A Alcoholism
L Leprosy
C Congenital disorders
A Acquired immunodeficiency syndrome (AIDS), Accidents
U Unsuccessful suicidal attempt
S Somatic diseases, Schizophrenia
E Epilepsy
S Speech disorders

O Osteomyelitis, Otitis media
F Functional psychiatric disorders
D Diabetes
I Iatrogenic disorders
S Septic arthritis
A Arthritis, Asthma
B Birth trauma, Brain damage
I Inflicting bodily injuries
L Loss of limbs
I Industrial accidents
T Traffic accidents
I Impairment of hearing and vision
E Earthquake
S Syphilis.

(Disability refers to inability to carry out certain activities considered normal for a human being, because of impairment. **C***ommunicable diseases,* **A***ccidents,* **P***oor quality of* **P***erinatal care and* **M***alnutrition (CAMP) are major causes of disability in the developing countries. Primary prevention is the most effective way of dealing with disability problems.)*

10. COLLECTIVE BARGAINING

"**BAN**" is Process of Collective Bargaining!

B Bargaining issues should be identify first
A *Agreement:* Reaching, ratifying and administration
N Negotiations (Advance preparation by both parties are essential).

(Collective bargaining is a technique for voluntary regulation of industrial relations. It is a process that determines relationship between the union and employer in regard to wages, working conditions and other benefits. One of the available methods for resolving disputes. Terms and conditions of employment are considered through collective bargaining and under which work is performed satisfactorily.)

11. ART OF LISTENING

"**LEADER**" must have Art of Listening!

(*Mnemonic:* LEADER)

L Look at the eyes of communicate
E Empathizing with the person speaking with you
A Ask questions related to topic of communication
D Do not change the topic
E Emotional status—check for it
R Responsive.

*(Listening is one of the most effective ways of communication. Majority of the managers do not know how to listen! Many of the problems that worry an administrator could have been totally avoided in the first place, if the administrator knew the art of listening. There are various ways in mastering the art of listening; "**LEADER**" is one of the easiest ways! Be good listener, have a better understanding and good relationships.)*

12. POWER

"**CLERK**" is the Main Sources/Base of Power!

C Coercive power, power to punishment, based on fear
L Legitimate power—power of position within the organization
E Expert power—personal power, based on one's skill and expertise
R Reward power, based on rewards—pay, promotion, recognition
Referent power—based on personal traits (Charisma)
K Knowledge is the power
Knowledge has to be improved, challenged, and increased constantly, or it vanishes.

(Power is easy to see but difficult to define. The capacity to produce effects on others. Successful leaders use a variety or even all of them. Motivation and resources are two essentials of power. The way we use power determines whether it is good or bad.)

13. LOGISTIC MANAGEMENT

Principles of Logistic Management:

(*Mnemonic:* MATERIALS)

M Materials and methods of handling
A Attitude towards improvements
T Time of delivery, transportation
E Economic order of quantity—right quantity
R Righteous principles, Right (People, place, price, procedures, packaging)
I Items/Intelligence materials
A At source
L Legal aspects
S Sources, System.

(These righteous elements can be achieved through various management techniques. Logistic management (LM) deals with supply of materials and allied activities in order to achieve maximum coordination and optimum expenditure on materials.)

14. PURCHASE

Types of Purchase

(*Mnemonic:* **CRIBS**, means things pilfered)

C Cash purchase/Bazaar purchase
R Reciprocity (It is a matter of top-management policy)
Rate contract—rate is fixed by tender, quantity not specified, reduce lead time
Running contract—minimum quantity is also specified
I Imprest purchase
B Blanket purchase
S Systemic purchase/stockless purchasing.

(Purchasing implies—procuring materials, supplies, machinery and services needed for production and maintenance of the concern. Purchasing and procurement are common functions. Purchasing refers to actual buying of materials and those activities associated with buying process.)

15. STANDARDIZATION

Benefits of Standardization

(*Mnemonic:* SIMPLE)

S Stock of spare parts reduced, seller-buyer relations improved

I Inventory reduction, items can be easily identified
Interchangeability of parts is assured
Inspection and QC burden can be reduced/eliminated

M Manager can focus on large quantity of fewer items
Minimizes obsolescence

P Paper work reduced

L Lead time reduction

E EOQ possible
Efficiency enhanced (handlers).

(Standardization is the orderly and systemic formulation, adoption, application and review of hospital standards. Process should be entrusted to a taskforce in the hospital. The role of standardization and variety reduction in inventory simplification has real significance in logistic management.)

16. OBSOLESCENCE

Reasons for Obsolescence:

(*Mnemonic:* STOCK)

S Standard items adopted, nonstandard items eliminated

T Technology/design changed

O Overstocking of spare parts

C Cannibalization of spare parts

K Keeping faulty store.

(Presence of obsolete items cannot be eliminated but can be controlled by better planning. Periodically analyze the movement of items and classify them as FSN. Nonmoving items subject to the XYZ analysis. List of "X" and nonmoving items is circulated to all departments before disposal. All pending orders for "X" and non-moving items are cancelled.)

17. INVENTORY CONTROL

Objectives of Inventory Control:

(*Mnemonic:* CMSO)

C Cost reduction
M Materials availability
S Stock minimize
O Optimal quantity.

(Inventory control is a scientific method of finding out how much stock should be maintained in order to meet the production demands and be able to provide right type of materials at right time in the right quantities and at competitive price. It aims at keeping track of inventories.)

18. EQUIPMENT FUNCTIONING

(*Mnemonic:* SERVE)

S Safety
E Effectiveness
R Reliability
V Validity
E Efficiency.

*(Discard any equipment when it became '**BERU**'–**B**eyond **E**conomic **R**epair, **U**nserviceable! Ensure that equipment should 'SERVE' properly in their day-to-day functioning. Equipment functioning effectively, safely and life-long, if maintain properly.)*

19. HOSPITAL

It Means

H House
O Of
S Sick
P People seeking
I Investigation
T Treatment either

A Ambulatory or
L Lying in bed.

(A hospital is an integral part of social and medical organization, the function of which is to provide for the population complete health care, both curative and preventive and whose outpatient services reach out to the family and its home environment; the hospital is also a center for the training of health workers and biosocial research—WHO definition of hospital.)

20. ASPECT OF CARE (ICU)

(*Mnemonic:* ASPECT OF CARE)

A Appropriateness of admission, ABG and other procedure: performance
S Staff satisfaction and complaints—evaluation, Statistical data: morbidity/mortality
P Performance of tracheotomy care, patient care in ventilator support
E Evaluation of nutritional needs, effects of medication monitoring, Errors
C CPR protocol development
T Timeliness of discharge
O Order (standard) compare with actual practice—assignments
F Failure of equipment assessed
C Care of patient should be evaluated
A Assessment of appropriate use of IV line
R Response time of clinicians
E Evaluation of patient satisfaction.

21. NURSING MANPOWER PLANNING

Nursing Manpower Planning Factors to be Considered Are:
(*Mnemonic:* BAD SAMPLE)

B Bed strength of the hospital
A Automation is the greatest industry (No one can stop it)
D Design and layout of the hospital

S Services available in the hospital
A Availability of technology and personnel
M Mechanization—centralization
P Pattern of assignment of nurse
L Labor-saving devices
E Emergency cases (types and numbers) coming to the hospital.

(All these factors should be considered for estimation of number of nurses required in a hospital. Nursing care depends on both quantity and quality of nursing personnel. Workload can be considered from three points of view: quality of nursing, characteristics of patients and schedule of nursing care. According to Nursing Committee (MOF, GOI), nurse-patient ratio should be 1:3 in hospital where nursing training is imparted, other hospitals should have a ratio of 1:5.)

22. FIRE TRIANGLE

Elements of Fire:

(*Mnemonic:* HOME)

H Heat
O Oxygen
M Materials, are fire triangle, and
E Essential elements to start a fire at anywhere.

(Fire is a triangle of three things, i.e. Heat, Material, and Oxygen. If any one out of these three elements is eliminated from the fire, the fire is automatically extinguished. DCP—dry chemical powder is the common fire extinguisher. Remember smoke is much more lethal than flame.)

23. *SIDDHA VAIDYA* SYSTEM

Siddha Vaidya System can be Effective in "**CHD**":

C Chronic diseases,
CNS disorders such as hemiplegia
H Heart diseases prevention
Hepatitis, Herpes-like viral infections

D Degenerative and autoimmune disorders such as rheumatoid arthritis.

(This is an ancient herbal medical system. Siddha vaids meticulously studied thousands of herbs for medicinal purposes. These herbal remedies have a tangible solution for various maladies. It forms a rational bridge between modern medicine and other alternative system of medicine. This system of medicine promises health and productive longevity.)

24. HOSPITAL FIRE

"**CSSD**" is the Most Frequent Causes of Hospital Fire

C Carelessness of CVS (contractors, visitors, staffs)
S Smoking
S Sometimes causes unknown
D Defective equipment, lighting, wiring.

(Carelessness is the common cause of fire in a hospital. Among all the potential hazards, fires pose a continual threat to the hospital. Patient safety is the primary concern and responsibility of hospital authority. All personnel working in the hospital should have basic knowledge about fire safety, fire fighting and rescue operation. Hospital should have own well laid-down fire manual.)

25. SELECTION

It means **RACE**

R Rejection
A Applicants by
C Choosing and
E Examining.

(The guiding policy in selection is the intention to choose the best suitable and qualified candidates. There is no standard selection process. Hospitals may follow different selection techniques. Government rules and regulation should be followed.)

26. DEMOGRAPHIC FACTORS

Demographic Factors in Epidemiological Studies:
(*Mnemonic:* MORALS)

M Marital status
O Occupation
R Race and religion
A Age
L Lifestyle
S Sex ratio.

(Demography is the scientific study of human population, deals with five demographic processes—maternity, mortality, marriage, migration and mobility (5Ms). Main sources of demographic statistics are population censuses, National sample survey, registration of vital events, and ad hoc demographic studies.)

27. FINANCIAL PLANNING

ABC of Financial Planning:

A *Accounting:* Data creation, collection, evaluation and reporting
B Budgeting
C Cost accounting and control of finance.

(Finance is the life of an organization. Good financial planning covers financial information, financial advice, cost analysis and cost control. Analysis and control of cost, budget, cost containment, financial statement analysis and control are some of the relevant tools for financial control in the hospitals.)

28. LABORATORY HAZARDS

Infectious Laboratory Hazards which can be Prevented:
(*Mnemonic:* H1, H2, and H3)

H1 HIV
H2 HBI
H3 HAI

(All laboratory personnel must be aware of common laboratory hazards. Carelessness is the single most important cause of any accidents. Laboratory specimens are potentially dangerous and may cause serious infections. When blood samples are taken, it must be assume that all patients are suffering from HIV or hepatitis, and universal precautions must be followed. No mouth pipetting is allowed in the laboratory. Take care while handling specimens.)

29. PRINCIPLES OF MANAGEMENT

(*Mnemonic:* POLICE)

P Planning
O Organizing
L Leading
I Integration
C Controlling
E Evaluating.

(Management principles and theories are mainly the product of rigorous scientific methodology. No management principles can be comprehended without proper scientific approach.)

30. RADIATION HAZARDS

ABC of Radiation Hazards (DELAYED EFFECTS)

A *Affection:* Almost all tissues and organs of the body
B Blood cancer
C Cancer
D Decreased of lifespan
E Epilation
F Fertility decreased
G Genetic mutation
H Hair falling

(Radiation injuries can arise from various sources like Alpha, Beta, Gamma and Neutrons. Radiation effects depend on type of cells of body affected, dose and source of radiation. The effect can be acute and chronic. Radiation protection and safety in all imaging techniques are of great concern to safeguard radiation hazards. Radiation protection facilities and disposal of radioactive waste are of paramount importance in radiotherapy center.)

31. MUDALIAR COMMITTEE

Recommendations of Mudaliar Committee

(*Mnemonic:* SPICE)

S Strengthening of PHU and district hospital
P Programs to eradicate communicable diseases at national level (Malaria, filariasis, tuberculosis, leprosy, cholera and smallpox)
I Insurance policy for all
C Central council of health making more effective
E Education in MEVA—Medical, Engineering, Veterinary, Agriculture.

32. DISTRICT PLANNER

Role and Responsibilities of District Planner

(*Mnemonic:* DISTRICT PLANNER CMO)

D District health manager, Disseminator, Decision maker
I Interpersonal contact role, Information processor
S Supervisor
T Team leader
R Resources provider
I Innovator
C Coordinator, communicator
T Themselves available to VIP
P Planner and promoter
L Leader and liaison
A Allocator of resources
N Negotiation

E Evaluator and facilitator
R *Role:* Legal, social, ceremonial
C Community contact maker
M Monitor and motivator
O Opinion leader.

33. BHORE COMMITTEE

Recommendations of Bhore Committee
(*Mnemonic:* HBP)

H Hospital, 30 bedded per 2 PHU
Health services demarcation into two parts—personal and impersonal
Hospital infrastructures for comprehensive health care
B Bhore, Sir Joseph is the Chairman of the committee
P Primary Health Unit—Supporting service unit, covering 20,000 to 40,000
Provision of preventive, promotive and curative services to all.

(The report of Bhore Committee was a landmark in the history of medical services. The term "comprehensive health care" was first used by Bhore Committee in 1946. By comprehensive services, Bhore Committee meant provision of integrated preventive, curative and promotional health services from "womb to tomb" to every individual residing in a defined geographical area. Committee suggested that comprehensive health care should replace the policy of providing more medical care. This concept formed the basis of national health planning in India and led to the establishment of a network of PHC and sub-centers.)

34. PREVENTIVE MAINTENANCE PROGRAM

ABC of Preventive Maintenance Program

A AC duct system periodic cleaning
B Building must be frequently inspected for loose slate, stone, plaster, and repair
C Ceiling and wall must maintain high hygienic standard
Cable: Avoid physical and mechanical pressure, select properly
D Doors and windows periodical checking

E Electrical equipment must be properly earthed

F Floor restores frequent cleaning

Fan and other electrical equipment must be switched off when not in use

G Gas connection must not be interchanged

Gas pipeline fault must attend immediately

H HVAC system periodical check up.

(Preventive maintenance is critical system maintenance to prevent possible breakdowns to a minimum. Parts which appear to be weak or worn out or likely to become defective are replaced before they actually fail or breakdown.)

35. HEALTH HAZARDS

Health Hazards Associated with Poor Hospital Waste Management

(*Mnemonic:* HAI)

H HAI to patient from poor infection control and poor waste management

A Antibiotics resistance due to change in microbial ecology

I Infection risk for handlers and general public

Injuries from sharp to all staff and waste handlers.

(Hospital waste: All waste generated, discarded and not intended for further use in the hospital. All hospital waste must manage in a scientific manner. All biomedical waste is hazardous. Improper handling, treatment and disposal of waste leads to serious problems. We have to preserve the earth for future generation.)

36. HOSPITAL WASTE MANAGEMENT

Managerial Issues for Effective Management of Hospital Waste

(*Mnemonic:* WASTED)

W Water supply, cleanliness, sanitation

A Awareness and education for proper segregation

S Switch to recycleable—minimize waste

T Tighten security to avoid illegal trading of the waste

E Explore non-burnt treatment
D Disinfection (chemical) at source.

(Hospital waste management is part of hospital hygiene and maintenance. It is a collective and shared responsibility of all. Waste management leads to clear and healthier surroundings.)

37. PATIENT'S RESISTANCE

"**DATE**" Decreased Patient's Resistance

D Diagnostic procedures, e.g. venipuncture, cardiac catheterization
A Aged persons, Ailments associated with AIDS, cancer, DM
T Therapeutic practice, e.g. indiscriminate use of antibiotics and steroids
E Endogenous infections.

(Decreased resistance of patients due to above-mentioned factors contribute to a great length on susceptibilities to hospital-acquired infection. Soundness of surveillance and control program depends on sound epidemiological knowledge.)

38. PERSONALITY DEVELOPMENT

Be "**PRACTICAL**" to Develop Personality

P People, Positive thinking
R Reading (Reader is the leader and Leader must be a reader!)
A Attempt/willing to change, Activity
C Circumstances
T Travel
I Involvement/experiences
C Challenges, Company you keep
A Attitude must be positive
L Listening and learning.

(Every person desires to improve his or her own personality. Personality goes beyond external appearance. It includes dispositions, traits, qualities, speech, and other things innate in the person. Improving your personality

takes a lot of work and dedication. Good physique, Pleasing manners, Personal and Professional integrity, Trustworthiness and reliability are attributes of a person with "pleasing personality".)

39. PATIENT DISSATISFACTION

BED can Dissatisfy the Patient

(*Mnemonic:* BED)

B Behavior of the nurses

E Environment of the hospital

D Dietary services.

(These three are the probable causes of patient dissatisfaction. Patient satisfaction is "hospital services and its perception by the patient" minus "patient expectations". Patient's satisfaction is an important indicator of quality of care being given to the patient. This is also necessary for survival and prosperity of the hospital. Satisfied patient acts as a virtual PRO of the hospital. To obtain the greatest degree of patient satisfaction, manage the "BED" properly!)

40. PERSON WITH DISABILITY

PWD can get Concession in AIR

(*Mnemonic:* AIR)

A Air traveling

I Income tax rebate

R Railway and road travel

Relaxation in age

Reservation in jobs (government sectors)

(PWD—Person with disability. Persons with disabilities Act, 1995 was passed by the parliament. The purpose is to fix responsibilities of Government to provide services, create facilities and give support to PWD.)

41. PREREQUISITES FOR BUDGETING

(*Mnemonic:* GOALS)

G Goal-clear identification of financial and service goals
O Organizational structure should be well designed
A All Accountability clearly defined, Accurate accounting system
L Limitation and value of budget must be understood by all
S Staff involvement and commitment of top management.

(Budgeting is fundamentally a people moving rather than paper moving process. All levels of management must understand its value and limitations.)

42. NURSING AUDIT

Nursing Audit: An Overview

(*Mnemonic:* PENS)

Nursing Audit, it means:

Periodic **E**valuation of **N**ursing **S**ervice.

P Pete Fisher RN has first time discussed it in 1953
E Evaluation is based on practical skills and qualification of
N Nursing staff, patient's satisfaction and turnover
S Service evaluation and improvement is the ultimate motto.

43. INPATIENT CARE

Factors Influencing Inpatient Care:

(*Mnemonic:* ABCDEFGHI)

A *Administrator:* Trained and experienced
B Beds utilization-effective use of beds
C Clinical and service facilities up to the mark
D Design and layout of the hospital
E Equipment, Education and training

F *Facilities:* Adequate space and pleasant environment
G General
H Hospital staff
I Index for arrangement of resources.

44. PRODUCTION PROCESS

3R for Production Process:
(*Mnemonic:* R1, R2, and R3)

R1 Resources (Men/Money/Material/Machine/Method)
R2 Ritual (Process/Techniques)
R3 Result (Output).

(Production is the process of producing goods or services which satisfy human wants. Productivity is nothing but ratio of input-output in respect to quality within time frame. Successful management creates a surplus through production process. The productivity of work is not the responsibility of the worker, but of the manager.)

45. CSSD

Functions of CSSD:
(*Mnemonic:* S1, S2, S3, S4, S5, S6, and S7)

S1 Supply of sterile items
S2 Sterilization processes are effectively controlled
S3 Sterilization quality
S4 Save the nursing time (most precious!)
S5 Safety of environment
S6 Safer and Standardized aseptic techniques
S7 Supply and equipment.

(Sterilization being one of the most essential services in the hospital requires the utmost consideration in planning. Concept of centralization increases efficiency, economy in use of equipment and ensures better supervision and control.)

46. OPERATING LIST

LIST should be ready for Operation:
(*Mnemonic:* LIST)

L Linen
I Instrument must be sterile and available
S Staff
T Time.

(Operating list is made for each operating room. Patient in the operating list must be operated at any cost. All administrative measures should be taken so that essential Linen, Instrument, Staff and Time are available for carrying out operation listed in the operating list.)

47. OT ASEPTIC STANDARDS

Maintenance and aseptic standards of OT:
(*Mnemonic:* ASEPTIC)

A AC duct and its filter should be checked thoroughly
S Sterilization of equipment and OT table should be ensured
Swab should be taken from various areas
E Electromedical equipment can fail at any time in spite of all precautions, thinks about alternatives.
P Persons having infections should not be allowed in OT
Pressure in various gases should be maintained all the time
T Time should be given for normal maintenance (one day/week)
Temperature and humidity check through gauges
I Infection rate should be constantly reviewed
C Compressed air, nitrous oxide, oxygen and suction are important manifold facilities.

48. GENERAL PRACTITIONERS

Areas in which GP Needs to be Involved

(*Mnemonic:* ABCDEFG)

A Ambulance services
B Basic health specialty
C Contraceptive services
D Drug supply (essential and rational)
E Education about community health
F First level referral healthcare
G GP provide services for personal healthcare.

49. PATIENT CARE

Essential Equipment for Patient Care

(*Mnemonic:* FACT OF BED)

F Fluids as per requirement
A Airways, Ambu bags
C Centralized O_2 and suction supply, Cardiac monitor
T Tables, Trollies, Trays, Tools, Table lamps (5Ts)
O *Others:* Glucometer, manometer
F Facilities for staffs
B Bags for resuscitation, Bandages and plaster
E Equipment for general Examination, ENT examination, laboratory, OT, ICU
ECG machine
D Drugs, Defibrillators.

50. ICU CLASSIFICATION

(*Mnemonic:* ABC, MNOP)

A Acute nursing care unit
B Burns unit
C Coronary ICU
M Medical and surgical ICU

N Neonatal ICU
O Obstetric ICU
P Pulmonary ICU
Pediatric ICU.

(ICU is a place and not a form of treatment. Above classification is based on type of patients admitted. All ICU can be of three types: open, closed and semi-closed unit. ICU of less than four beds and less than 200 cases per year with an average occupancy of less than 75% is considered uneconomical.)

51. PEDIATRIC ICU

Additional **SPACE** requirement for PICU:
(*Mnemonic:* SPACE)

S Space at each bed side
Separate space for visitors
P Provision for formula preparation
A Allowance of space equal to adult
C Cabinet for toys and games
E Examination and treatment room, minimum floor area 120 SF with Washing fixture, storage facilities, desk and a counter.

52. ENVIRONMENT

SPECIAL Environments, it means:
(*Mnemonic:* SPECIAL)

S Social environment
P Political environment
E Ethical environment
C Cultural environment
I International environment
A Activist, environmental protection
L Legal environment.

(Environment: The sum total of all the conditions and elements that make up the surroundings and influence the development of an individual.)

53. DISASTERS: BE PREPARED!

ABCD of Disasters:

(*Mnemonic:* ABCDEF)

A Accidents
B Bomb blast
C Cyclone
D Deluge
E Earthquake
F Fire and Flood.

(India is a disaster prone country. Disaster management means a planned and systemic approach towards understanding and solving problems in the wake of disaster. To understand the disaster is first important aspects to manage the disaster. Pre-planning prevents poor performance. Human life is major concern. Remember 3D for disaster: Damage and ecological disruption, Deterioration of health and health services, Death.)

54. TYPES OF DISASTERS

(*Mnemonic:* FIRE)

F Flood and fire,
Failure of structure
I *Internal disaster:* HBP
R Radiation release,
Rail/road and air accidents
E Earthquake
H Hot war/war like situation (external)
B Bomb blast
P Power/water/sewerage disruption
Patient/visitors agitations.

55. HOSPITAL AREAS

Security sensitive areas of the hospital:

POLICE is a security sensitive area of the hospital.

P Pediatric unit, pharmacy, parking
O Office of medical records

L Lock restrict movement of people in these areas
I Infant unit
C Cash handling unit, Computer, Cafeteria (3Cs)
E Emergency department.

(Strict and efficient security is essential for these areas.)

56. HOSPITAL
(*Mnemonic:* HOSPITAL)

H Health services and social organization
O Organization of various diversity and dual authority
S Service and community oriented
P Patient care focused
I Inpatient facilities
T Training of staff, as well as
A Ambulatory and emergency services
L Licensed by appropriate authority.

(Today hospital means an institution in which sick or injured persons are treated. Medical dictionary defines a hospital as, "an institution for the care, cure and treatment of the sick and wounded, for the study of diseases and for the training of doctors and nurses. Hospital should be easily accessible to the public and planned in accordance with norms, standards and prevailing laws.)

57. DISASTER CLASSIFICATION
Manmade Disaster:
(*Mnemonic:* WARRENT)

W Ware fare—bomb blast
A Accidents—building collapse
R Riots and demonstration
R Refugees
E Else, fire and food poisoning

N Nonconventional warfare

T Technological failure, Terrorism, Transportation calamities.

Natural Disaster: A to F

A Avalanches

B Biological disaster, insect swarm

C Cyclones, Cold spells

D Droughts

E Earthquake, epidemics of communicable diseases

F Flood.

58. THREATS AND VULNERABILITIES

Common Threats and Vulnerabilities in the Hospital
(*Mnemonic:* CID FOR THREATS)

C Civil disturbances, Crime-white collar crime

I Infant abduction, Information losses

D Drug abuse, Disaster, Damage of property

F Firing

O Others manmade disasters

R Rape (sexual assault)

T Threat to medical and nonmedical personnel

H Hazards to health, hygiene, safety

R Robbery upon staff

E Employees and patient property loss

A Arson, Anti-national activities

T Theft (external and internal)

S Strikes, Sexual assaults.

59. EQUIPMENT DISPOSAL

Any one of the Following Measures can be Adopted:
(*Mnemonic:* SCRAP)

S Selling to the scrap dealers
Sell to others hospitals

C Circulate within the hospital's department
R Return to the vendors, if he is willing to accept it
A Auction
P Put to end by local destruction.

(Any of the above procedure can be adopted for disposal of equipment after condemnation.)

60. CONDEMNATION

Criteria for Condemnation:
EQUIPMENT:

1. FUNCTIONAL	**2. NON-FUNCTIONAL (BERO)**
1a. Hazardous	2a. Beyond economic repair (BER)
1b. Obsolete	2b. Obsolete
1c. No longer required	

(Condemnation committee decides whether or not an equipment should be condemned and disposed off on the basis of history sheet and recommendations by user department. For condemnation of costly equipment, a special condemnation board may formed.)

61. DIETARY SERVICE

Functions of Hospital Dietary Service:
(*Mnemonic:* DIET)

D Diet counseling
I Inpatient and commercial catering
E Education staff and patients
T Training and research activities
Therapeutic diets: Planning, preparation, distribution.

(The dietary service of a hospital is an important therapeutic tool. Aim should be to produce well-cooked appetizing and nutritious food as economically as possible. Hospital kitchen alone could be responsible for spreading the diseases, if hygienic conditions are not maintained and also shortening patient stay in the hospital, if rendered properly.)

62. GOOD HOUSEKEEPING

Functions of Good Housekeeping

(*Mnemonic:* CASE)

C Cost of care reduced
A ALS reduced (Average Length of Stay)
S Suffering of patient reduced
E Enhances public relation and patient satisfaction.

(Housekeeping is defined as—the provision of a clean, comfortable and safe environment for the patients and public in a hospital set-up. This is a non-revenue-producing service department in the hospital. A poorly run department results in money needlessly spent and creates a negative impression on patients, visitors and staff, which will adversely affect their perception of the quality of care provided by the hospital.)

63. SLIP HAZARDS

(*Mnemonic:* FIND TQM)

F Friction need
I Indoor-outdoor use
N Nature of areas
D Durability
T Traffic need (special)
Q Quality of surface
M Method of quality to be employed.

(To prevent slip hazards, variable elements to considered in selection process are mainly related to use base.)

64. ICU STAFFING PATTERN

Staff Requirement for 8 Bedded ICU:

(*Mnemonic:* DR CP DAS)

D Director of ICU (1)
R Registrar/SHO (on rotation) (4)
C Consultant (1)

P Peon (1)
D Domestic staff (4)
A Administrator of ward (2)
S Secretary (1)
Sister (42), Charge nurse-4, Trained nurse-32, Nurses in training-6 (Total staff: 56—direct requirements for provision of constant medical care.)

65. GOAL

Goal must be "SMART".
It means:

S Specific
M Measurable
A Achievable/actionable
R Relevant
T Time bound.

(Goals are aimed at achieving the vision. They should be achievable in short span of time and represent what you can see and reach. Clarification of goals then sets the agenda for the strategies (how) that are necessary to achieve those goals, to drive those goals forward. The strategies then need to be broken down into very specific action plans. Goals are not constrained by time or existing resources.)

66. PROCUREMENT

Six Factors Governing Procurement:
(*Mnemonic:* PQRST)

P Price and place
Q Quality and quantity
R Right choice criteria (Righteous criteria)
S Source
T Time factor (Right time delivery).

(Procurement is broader in scope and includes purchasing, storage and all activities related to receiving inbound materials.)

67. SEWAGE

SEWAGE is Fundamental Facilities!

S Sewage disposal
E Electricity
W Water supply
A Air conditioning
G Gases and air
E Elevator.

68. BLOOD DONOR

Blood Donor Selection/Rejection Criteria:
(*Mnemonic:* WHAT IS BP)

W Weight more than 45 kg
H Hemoglobin more than 12.5 g%, Healthy person
A Age between 18 and 60 years
T Temperature not exceed 37.5°C
I Immunizations? Infections, Intoxication of drugs, alcohol
S Systemic examination should be normal
B *Blood pressure:* Systolic: 100–150 mm Hg, Diastolic: 60–90 mm Hg
P *Pulse:* 60–90 per minute.

(Donor recruitment and bleeding donors are the most important managerial issue for a blood bank. If only 1% of the population donate one unit of blood per year the nation's required blood needs would be met. Organized institutions or groups are rich sources of qualified blood donors. Greater stress has been laid on voluntary donors; professional donors are banned by laws.)

69. NURSING ACTIVITIES

"**CARE**" is one of the prime Nursing Activities.
(*Mnemonic:* CARE)

C Care of the patient is the core activity

A Administration
R Records and reports maintenance, routine information
E Educational aspect,
Environment maintenance.

70. NURSE-PATIENT RATIO

Nurse-Patient ratio as per SIU norms:
(I DO ON CAI => 1:1, 1:2, 1:3, 1:4, and 1:5)

I	ICU	1:1
D	Delivery room	1:1
O	OT major	1:1
O	OT minor	1:2
N	NICU and Burns	1:2
C	Casualty	1:3
A	Ambulatory (opd)	1:4
I	Inpatient (ward)	1:5

(SIU—Staff Inspection Unit has recommended nursing norms in 1991–92. As per these norms, nurse-patient ratio is 1:3 for teaching hospital and 1:5 for nonteaching hospital. Most of the hospital including central government hospital is following the SIU norms.)

71. COST CONTAINMENT

Doctors Reduce Bills by Cutting Down **DILS**!

D *Drugs:* Cutting down unnecessary drugs and therapies
I *Investigations:* Cutting down unnecessary investigations
L *Length of stay:* Cutting down length of stay
S *Supplies, services and (re)sources:* Economic use of it.

(Motivate all the staffs to contain cost. HIS, personnel data and quality control are basic requirement for effective cost control activities. Key to success in cost containment lies in cost awareness, cost monitoring and cost management.)

72. HOSPITAL INFORMATION SYSTEM (HIS)

(*Mnemonic:* COST)

C Control function, e.g. cost control, medical audit
O Operational planning, e.g. budgeting, purchasing
S Strategic planning, e.g. services to be offered, image improvement plan
T Transaction process, e.g. patient billing, inventory control.

(The framework of the hospital information system should be so organized that there is rapid and regular feedback of information, related to the quality of care rendered by clinical departments and also overall performance of all services.)

73. SKILLS OF AN ADMINISTRATOR

(*Mnemonic:* LINC)

L Leadership skill
I Interpersonal skill (human relations)
N Negotiation skill
C Conflict management.

74. STORES SAFETY AND SECURITY

LIST—for Security and Safety Aspect of Stores

L Locking and
Labeling properly
I Inventory control measure,
Indent form must be printed
S Security staff should be sufficient
T Transportation of materials.
(Movement of men must be manage by security.)

75. FIRE EXTINGUISHER

"**PASS**" for Proper and Effective use of Fire Extinguisher

P Pull the pin
A Aim low

S Squeeze the handle

S Sweep from side to side.

(Extinguishment is the last resort to fire safety program. Extinguishers can be used according to grade of fire. Pressurized water and CO_2 can be used on class A and class B, C fires respectively. DCP (dry chemical powder) and Halon are commonly used fire extinguishers for all types of fires. Suppression of fire can be achieved by manually or automatic extinguishing system.)

76. DEMANDS OF PATIENTS

Patients want "KHUSHI" rather than "KITS":

KHUSHI, means:

K Kindness

H Honesty

U Understanding

S Sympathy

H Hearty feeling

I Interest.

KITS, means:

K Knowledge

I Intelligence

T Training

S Skills.

77. PHC STAFFING PATTERN

STAFF AT NEW PHC:

(*Mnemonic:* MD AT NEW PHC)

M Medical officer (1)

D Driver (1)

A Assistant, health male (1)

T Technician (1)

N Nurse as a midwife (1)

E Educator, health (1)
W Worker, female health (1)
P Pharmacist (1)
H Health assistant (female) (1)
C Class-4, Clerk-upper and lower division (2).

78. NATIONAL AIDS CONTROL PROGRAM

ABC of AIDS Control Program

(*Mnemonic:* ABCDEF)

A AIDS control program integrated with STD control program
B Blood safety program was started in 1989, to ensure safety of blood
C Condom program, Control of STDs.
D Data collection—Surveillance is being done through HIV sentinel surveillance at selected centers.
E Education, information and communication
F For high-risk behavior (target)—behavioral modification.

(Infection with HIV is a global problem. HIV infection is spreading from high risk to low risk groups and from urban to rural areas. The program was started in 1987. NACO was established under Ministry of Health and Family Welfare for effective implementation and monitoring of the program.)

79. MINIMUM NEED PROGRAM

Components of Minimum Need Program

(*Mnemonic:* WHERE IS NRHM)

W Water supply
H Health services to rural areas
E Electrification, environmental improvement of urban slums
R Roads for rural development
E Elementary education and education to adult
I Improve environment of urban slum
S Sanitation
N Nutrition programs

R Rural and domestic cooking
H Housing assistance to landless laborers
M Mechanism-system of public distribution.

(NRHM: National Rural Health Mission)
(The program was launched in 1974–78 with objective to provide certain basic minimum needs and thereby improve the living standards of the people. Delivery of rural health services through three-tier system is the main component.)

80. INTEGRATED CHILD DEVELOPMENT SCHEME (ICDS)

ICDS Packages of Services:
(*Mnemonic:* IT SNEH)

I Immunization progams
T Treatment of minor illness
S *Service:* Supportive and referral
N Nutritional supplements, IFA tablets (Iron and Folic Acid)
E Education to women and children regarding health and nutrition
H Health check up.

(ICDS was launched in 1975. It is a multisectoral program and involves several government departments. Children below 6 years, adolescent girls, expectant and nursing mothers and women in reproductive age group are main beneficiaries.)

81. ROLE OF HOSPITAL IN RCH PROGRAM

(*Mnemonic:* RCH-I, or RICH)

R Referral system and research activity—clinical and operational research
C Clinical skill based training to health personnel
H Health education in hospital
I Information about "BEDS", means—Beds, Epidemics, Death, Surveillance

82. ROLE OF HOSPITAL IN NHP

(*Mnemonic:* ESCORT)

E Ensure care of case referred from periphery
S Sentinel surveillance
C Carry out survey and screening for early detection
O Organizing health education activity
R Rehabilitation services
T Training of manpower in clinical and diagnostic aspect.

83. FIRE FIGHTING

Essential Steps when Fire Breaks Out:
(*Mnemonic:* SAVE)

S Save patient or persons if in immediate danger
A Alarm, activate the nearest alarm, dial security
V *Vent:* Closed doors and windows to contain fire
E Evacuate and extinguish.

(Prompt action is must. Delay in action can make big difference, may result in tragic disaster. A step in time saves both lives and property.)

84. NATIONAL MALARIA ERADICATION PROGRAM

SLIDE is a Major Activity of NMEP

S Surveillance by blood smears collection fortnightly
L Laboratory service at PHC level
I Insecticide spray
D Drug distribution center established
E *ETC:* Established fever treatment depot
Treatment radical and presumptive
Control and containment of *Plasmodium falciparum.*

85. STD MANIFESTATIONS

(*Mnemonic:* PUS)

P Pain at lower abdomen
U Ulcers at genital, urethral and vaginal discharge
S Swelling at inguinal region.

(Early diagnosis and treatment of STD is now recognized as one of the major strategies to control spread of HIV infection. HIV is transmitted more easily in presence of STD. Patient with STD form special group for health education and counseling.)

86. TOTAL QUALITY MANAGEMENT

ABC of Total Quality Management:

(*Mnemonic:* ABC)

A Aimed at long-term success through customer satisfaction
And benefits to all employees and to the society
B Based on participation of all its members
C Central approach is quality.

(Feigenbaum developed the concept of Total Quality Control [TQC]. This concept has laid down the foundation for Total Quality Management [TQM]).

87. QUALITY MANAGEMENT SYSTEM

Aims of QMS:

(*Mnemonic:* QMS)

Q Quality of service
M Management assurance through effective control process
S Service conforms to customer's requirement.

(Management system to direct and control the organization with regard to quality. Quality management is a means of ensuring efficiency and effectiveness. Quality management is a mandatory requirement in certain countries. Quality management programs promote satisfaction to both patients and staffs.)

88. SOCIAL AGENTS

Social Agents which are Known to Aid Causation of Disease:
(*Mnemonic:* SAD)

S Smoking, social isolation
A Abuse of alcohol
D Drugs, deprivation.

(The first link in the chain of disease transmission is a disease agent. It is also necessary to consider social agents of disease. These social agents also make sad to the society.)

89. MANPOWER PLANNING AND PROGRAMS

(*Mnemonic:* CREATS)

C Career planning
R Recruitment, Retirement, and Replacement
E Efficiency investigation
A Appraisal and development
T Training
S Selection.

(Remember, Manpower is the main power in an organization.)

90. OBJECTIVE

(*Mnemonic:* FORAM)

F Feasible/flexible
O Observable
R Relevant, Realistic
A Achievable
M Measurable.

(Objective may be defined as the specific goals or targets to be accomplished, as for example, cost reduction, increase in productivity, personal development, and social responsibility. It ensures performance control and adds to the planning. It should be backed by suitable sub goals.

It is a measurable state of accomplishment aimed towards the goal. The objective should include a description of "what" outcome is desired, "when" it is expected, and "where" it will take place.)

91. PLANNING

Plan must be "**PERFECT**".

(*Mnemonic:* PERFECT)

P Participation and pass on to all concerned
E End result desired
R Realistic
F Flexible, Forecasting is inherent
E Economy of performance assured
C Comprehensible, continually updated
T Time phase.

(Planning is a projected or predetermined course of action designed to achieve a specific goal or objective. Pre-planning prevent poor performance. Planning determines What? When? Where? How? Why? And by whom? Things will be done. It involves "decision making for future events".
Many managers are powerful in making plans but very poor in its implementation. Plan without implementation has no value, merely waste of time and other resources.)

92. MATERIAL MANAGEMENT PROCESS

(*Mnemonic:* PRICES)

P Planning and demand forecasting, Purchasing
R Receipt
I Inspection, Issue, Inventory control
C Condemnation and disposal
E Eliminating losses and pilferage
S Store.

93. ORGANIZATION STRUCTURE

ABCD of Organization Structure:

(*Mnemonic:* ABCD)

A Authority and responsibility
B *Body:* Governing and executive
C Coordination, Centralized/decentralized
Command and control (unity of command, span of control)
D Delegation
(Structure defines formal relationships of the people in the organizations).

94. PURCHASING PROCESS

(*Mnemonic:* ISI)

I Inviting tenders
S *Specification:* Drawing up, *Statement:* Comparative
Shortlisting
I Issuing purchase order.

(Purchasing is the acquisition of the property and materials needed in administration.
Ultimate aim: Right quality, right quantity, right prices, right source and at right time to the right place.)

95. PUBLIC HEALTH SERVICES

Public Health Services: Concerned Issues

(*Mnemonic:* MCHs)

M Maternal and child health
C *Communicable diseases:* Prevention and control
H "HOPE" of Health, it means
Hazards, ***O***ccupation, ***P***lanning, and ***E***ducation
S Sanitation and statistics.

(Public health is a science which involves methods to prevent diseases and improve the well being of the general public. Presently, public health has been replaced by community health due to its wide all embracing

community organized efforts for maintaining, protecting, preventing and promoting health of the people.)

96. REGIONALIZATION OF HEALTH CARE

(*Mnemonic:* DECENTRALISATION)

D District is viable unit, Decentralization of healthcare
E Elements of regionalization
C Central to regionalization
E Economy and ecology are criteria for demarcation of region
N NHP sometime creates problems in regionalization
T Three-tier system in healthcare
R Regionalization of healthcare which closely the regionalization of administration machinery
A A body classified in successively subordinate grade—hierarchy
L Level of care at PHC, CHC, and DH are known as primary, secondary and tertiary care
I Implementation of any program always needs careful planning and dedicated personnel
S Structuring of authority and responsibility
A Aim is to provide comprehensive health care at defined geographic areas
T TP and GP are viable for local administration
I Integrated authority system for coordination
O Overall benefits of regionalization
N Nodal regions.

97. PROGRAM EVALUATION AND REVIEW TECHNIQUE (PERT)

(*Mnemonic:* PERT)

P Project plan presentation in a Network form
PSM technique (Planning, scheduling, monitoring)
E Elements are events and activities
Evaluation and checking system are built on it.
R Resources clarification to complete the task on time.
T *Time:* Event network analysis.

98. LAW RELATED TO HOSPITAL

(*Mnemonic:* PHORENSIC MEDICINE)

P Pharmacy Act, 1948, Poison Act, 1919,
Payment of Gratuity Act, 1972, Payment of Wages Act, 1936
H Homoeopathy Central Council Act, 1972
Human Organs Transplantation Act, 1994
O Opium Act, 1978
R Registration of Society Act, 1860
E Employment Exchange Act, 1959
N Nursing Council Act, 1947
S Sex Determination Act, Sexual Harassment Act
I Indian Medical Council Act, 1956,
Indian Medical Central Council Act, 1970
Industrial Dispute Act, 1947
C Consumer Protection Act, 1986
M Medical Termination of Pregnancy Act, 1971
Minimum Wages Act, 1984
Maternity Benefit Act, 1961
E Employees Provident Fund Act, 1952
D Drug and Cosmetic Act, 1940
Dangerous Drug Act, 1930
Drug Act, 1950
I Income Tax Act, 1961
C Company Act, 1956
I Industrial Dispute Act, 1947
N Notification of Vacancies Act, 1959
E Equal Remuneration Act.

(In addition to above Acts and Rules framed thereunder, there are many decisions of the Supreme Court, High Courts and local self-government (Corporation) which have bearing on the functioning of the hospitals. Hospital Administrator must be conversant with them.)

99. HIGH-RISK FACTORS

MEDICATIONS are the high-risk factors

M Medications
E Environmental pollution
D Dietary factor, Diabetes
I Infectious agents
C Cholesterol level elevated
A Alcohol, Accident, Addiction
T Type A personality, Tension
I Ionizing radiation
O Obesity
N Non use of seat belts
S Smoking, Sedentary life, Speed, Stress, Solar radiation (5S).

100. NATIONAL HEALTH POLICY

(*Mnemonic:* UNESCO)

U Universal Immunization Programmes (UIP)
N Nutrition programs
E Environmental protection
S Sanitation and safe water supply
School health programs
C Child health services—MCH services
Contamination and adulteration of food and drugs
O Occupational health services.

(These are priority/problematic areas of National Health Policy which require urgent attention.)

101. STRESS MANAGEMENT STRATEGIES (SMS)

(*Mnemonic:* DISTRESS)

D Delegation
I Individual stress reduction workshop, Information and help from others

S Supervisor training program
T Time management
R Role analysis techniques, relocation of job, recreational programme
E Employee assistance program
S Sport and gym facilities for health maintenance
S Stress management program
Specialized advised for career path.

(Stress is a reality of our everyday life. There are both eustresses and distresses that come from our work and non-work lives. One of the major sources of job stress is the job itself. Interpersonal relationship and problems in personal life can cause job stress. 80% of all modern diseases have their origins in stress. It is important for individuals to optimally manage their stress to operate as fully functioning human beings.)

102. SYSTEM CHANGE

"**QUEST**" for Using Data to Stimulate System Change!

Q *Question:* What is the actionable question?
U *Understanding:* What are the relevant variables?
Measures and analyses to address the question?
E Efficiently and effectively analyze the data
S Synthesize and summarize results in a relevant manner for each audience
T Tell the story and finally,
Take an action.

(Change simply means the alteration of status-quo. Even in the most successful and stable system, change is necessary for survival. An organization must be ready for change and top management should inform the employees about the change.)

103. PRIMARY HEALTH CARE

ABC of Primary Health Care

(Principles of PHC)

A Accessible, acceptable, affordable and appropriate technology, (A4)
B Base on practical

C Community participation
D Distribution of health services should be equitable that is
E Equity in health care
F Focus on prevention.

(A new approach to health care came into existence in 1978, followed an international conference at Alma Ata. Primary healthcare is equally valid for all countries.)

104. COST CONTROL

(Components of Cost Control Activity)
"**QWERY**" for any Cost Control Activity!
(*Mnemonic:* QWERY)

Q Quality ensuring
W Waste minimization
E Efficiency maximization
R Resources used optimally
Y Why cost control is so IMP-Improving and Measuring Performance?

(Cost control is defined as any activity that aims at defining, measuring and improving level of performance. Cost control programmers are not aimed at entailing the quality or quantity of services provided to the patients. They are aimed at increasing performance efficiency of the healthcare team.)

105. QUALITIES OF HOSPITAL ADMINISTRATOR

Hospital Administrator should be **DIPLOMATIC**
(*Mnemonic:* DIPLOMATIC)

D Diplomatic
I Intelligent judge of human nature (human skill)
P Pleasing personality
L Leadership skills
O Organizing capacity, Orderly appearance
M Man with fine business senses, mentally robust
A Ability to withstand frequent adverse criticism

T Tactful, Take the job seriously
I Infinitely patient
C Cordially working with everyone, Credit giver,
Conceptual skills.

106. HOSPITAL STRUCTURE

These Criteria should be Considered for Hospital Structure.
(To avoid chaos in the hospital, consider "**CHAOS**")

C Communication's problems and ensure effective
Communication at all levels
H Hospital's size, shape, location and capacity
A Administrative structure accordingly
Authority: Limitation of functional authority
O Objective of the hospital and types of activities to reach them
S *Specialization:* Its benefits and maximization.

(Medical, Nursing and Administrative department are three common points of hospital structure.)

107. TYPES OF HOSPITALS

(Types of Hospital According to Hospital Directory)
SIR TG is a teaching hospital at Bhavnagar.

S Specialized hospital
I Isolation hospital
R Rural hospital
T Teaching hospital
G General hospital.

(Directory of hospital, defined the hospital as an institution which is operated for the medical, surgical and/or obstetrical care of inpatient and which is treated as a hospital by the central or state government or local bodies or licensed by the appropriate authority.)

108. UNICEF

Functions of UNICEF:
(*Mnemonic:* WHEN GOBI)

W *Welfare:* Child and family
H Health
E *Education:* Formal and informal
N Nutrition programs
G Growth charts to monitor child development
O ORS for ORT (Oral rehydration solution for oral rehydration therapy to mild and moderate dehydrations)
B Breastfeeding promotion network
I Immunization against infectious diseases.

(United Nations International Children's Emergency Fund is a specialized agency of United Nations, established in 1946, for rehabilitation of children in war-ravaged countries with headquarters in New York and regional office at New Delhi.)

109. SITE SELECTION

For Site Selection, **REAL** Factors are:

R Resources availability (sewage line, electricity, and water)
E Environment (plenty of fresh air, sunlight, free from pollution)
Easy reach of the community
A Areas and Accessibility
L Land required (100 Square feet per bed, *Total covered area:* 1000 SFPB).

(Hospital site should be large enough for future expansion. Hospital should be planned at least 5–10 years ahead. Area and land requirement depend on bed strength and services provided by the hospital. As per National Institute of Health, New Delhi, the members of the community should be able to reach the hospital within a travel time of 30 minutes.)

110. ARCHITECTURAL DRAWINGS

Types of Architectural Drawings

(*Mnemonic:* SAME)

S *Structural drawing:* Structural sections, slab, beam, column

A Architectural drawings (ABCDEFGHI)

A	Actual drawing showing
B	Building location and site plan
C	Consecutive floor plans
D	Doors and windows schedules
E	Elevator
F	Finishes
G	General and wall sections
H	Highways (road/walkways)
I	Interior/exterior details.

M *Mechanical drawings:* Concerned with **WAVES**

Water supply service (*Sources:* Underground, hot/cool)

Air conditioning

Ventilating,

Equipment/fixture schedules,

Sewage system, Storm water

E Electrical drawing (EEEEEE)—6E

Entry of electricity into building

Electrical feeder

Electric panel location

Electrical equipment, and related items

Electrical shielding (static)

Electrical system for lighting, intercommunication and fire alarms.

(Architectural drawing is the collective efforts of an architect which represent clinical, administrative and technical (CAT) requirements of the hospital into architectural and engineering reality.)

111. COMMUNICATION

Elements of Communication
(Communication Model/Process)
(*Mnemonic:* SENDER)

S **Sender/Sources** starts communication process

E **Encoding** (sender translates information into a series of symbols)

N **Noise** (any factor that interfaces with communication)

D **Decoding** (receiver interprets message and translates into meaningful information)

E **Encoded** message transmitted through proper channels

R **Receiver**, who receives the message.

(Communication is a process of transmitting information (PTI) from sender to receiver resulting in common understanding to all. It is important for internal functioning of the organization and for the interaction with external environment. It is impossible to have human relations without communication. Effective communication is the foundation of sound management. An average executive spends almost 70% of his working time in communication.)

112. GENERAL STANDARDS

ABC of General Standards for Details and Finishes

A **Air** and light should enter into the rooms

Architectural finishes should be of high quality

B **Building** design should ensure noise control

C **Circulation** areas should not be < 30% of total floor area

Corridor width should be 8 feet and as straight as possible

Ceiling height at least 8 feet and acoustically treated to reduce sound transmission

Clinics area, toilet should be provided within clinics

Conductive flooring should be avoided in the areas where flammable anesthetic agents are stored.

Ceilings and walls in CSSD, OT, labor room, and nursery should be monolithic from wall to wall without open joints.

D **Doors** should be operable on both sides on OT, only inside at other place
Doors width to patient room preferably 1.16 meter
Doors should not swing into corridor
Dark room is too small (6 × 6) feet

E **Electrical** outlets should be provided on the walls of the corridor.
Expression joints should have non-metallic beading finish.
Expansion joints should be made flush with floor to facilitate the smooth movements of trolley, wheelchairs, and stretchers
Elevator:
- ! Location should be decided by maximum concentration of traffic
- !! Minimum two elevators for any multi-storied building
- !!! Elevator call buttons and controls should not be activated by heat/smoke
- !!!! Elevator doors should not be open into the main lobby.

F **Floor** should not be hard type; height should not be < 3 meter
Flooring in the sanitary blocks should be made with marbles

G **General** OPD, *waiting area:* 8–10 sq.ft per patient visit.

H **Handrails** should be provided on both sides of the stairways at the height of 3 feet
Heat generating areas should be insulated and ventilated properly.

113. ELECTRICAL STANDARDS

Electrical Standards—General Consideration
(*Mnemonic:* ELECTRICALS)

E **Electrical** supply must be dependable and uninterruptible
Electrical supply may be at high or low voltage depending on load
Electrical power is distribute at 415/20V using a separate protective conductor.

L **Lamps**, luminaries, lighting and levels of illumination should be as per NEC.
Lighting distribution boards should be located on the same floor

E **Electrical** call and signal systems should be provided in the hospitals
Emergency lighting of three types (A/B/C) to be provided
Electrical equipment must be earthed properly

C **Cables** are preferably underground.

T **Three** types of power supply (standby/safety/special safety)
Telephone cables should be brought into the building basement
Telephone cables and power cables should be laid down separately to prevent mechanical damage, chemical actions or heat

R **Rigid** nonmetallic conducts of ample size are generally used for concealed wiring.

I **Interconnecting** telephones should be provided to all the areas.

C **Circuit** breaker (MCB) for power and lighting circuits to protect small wires and flexible cords.

A **Air** circuit breakers are used on secondary of the transformers.
Alarm system: NBC guidelines should be followed

L **Lift** should conform to IS 3534.

S **Socket** outlets should be provided in all areas where plug in service is required.
Safety type sockets should be provided in the pediatrics and psychiatric wards.
Six sockets in OT and DR (delivery room)
Socket *per bed:* Minimum three
(*NBC:* National Building Code, *MCB:* Miniature Circuit Breaker).

114. THEORY X VERSUS THEORY Y

WARS against Theory X and Theory Y

		Theory X	Theory Y
W	*Work:*	People dislike works	People enjoy work like play
A	*Ambition:*	Lack of ambition	Highly ambitious, innovative, creative
R	*Responsibility:*	Avoid responsibility	Accept responsibility
S	*Supervision:*	Needs close supervision	self-controlled

(McGregor's Theory X and Theory Y are two sets of assumptions about the nature of people. These two sets of assumptions are fundamentally opposite. X people are pessimistic, static and rigid, while Y people are optimistic, dynamic and flexible.)

115. ORGANIZATIONAL BEHAVIOR

(Elements of Organizational Behavior)

STEP of Organizational Behavior

S Structure (formal relationships of the people in the organization)

T *Technology:*

Affects organization structure

Determination of objectives often depends on it,

Provide extra resources to do productive work, but restrict the people.

E *Environment:*

All organization operates within external environment, which is a part of larger system that contains other elements such as government, family, and others, all of these mutually influence each other in a complex system.

P *People:*

Make up the internal and social system of the organization

They work to achieve their objectives

Without people, no organizations have reasons to exist

People are the most valuable and the greatest assets of the organization.

(OB is study of human behavior in the organization.)

116. PERSONALITY

Personality Factors in Organizations:

(*Mnemonic:* LEARNS MIND)

L Locus of control

E Extroversion, Ethic orientation

A Ambiguity, tolerance for it, Authoritarianism

R Risk propensity

N Need pattern

S Self-concept, Self-esteem

M Machiavellianism

I Introversion

N Nothing but type A and type B personality

D Dogmatism

SHE determines personality:

Situation,

Heredity, and

Environment.

(Personality is the sum total of characteristics and appearances that distinguish from all others. Our personality traits determine how we react in specific situations and how we adjust to our environment. Character is the most important part of the personality rather than outward appearance.)

117. JOB SATISFACTION

6P For Job Satisfaction

P1 Positive feelings that persons have towards their jobs

P2 Pay scale

P3 Promotion (Promotional avenue having some motivational value)

P4 Place

P5 Policies

P6 Procedures.

(There is no standard definition of job satisfaction. Organizational and personnel are two variables that determine the job satisfaction. Higher the level of job, greater is the satisfaction. It is a general attitude towards work by an individual worker.)

118. GROUP

What Makes People Join Groups?

To fill **GAPS**, people join the groups!

G Goal achievement

A Affiliation

P Power and prestige

S Status, Security, and Self-esteem (3S).

(Human behavior comprises individuals and individuals form groups. They live in groups, move in groups, and work in groups. Groups are important. Groups are dynamics. Individual behavior is influenced by group behavior. Group behavior affects productivity. Groups may be formal, informal or task type.)

119. SENSITIVE AREAS OF THE HOSPITAL

CORE (sensitive) Areas of the Hospital

C Casualty department
O Outpatient department
R Reception and Registration
E Enquiry office.

120. POLITICAL BEHAVIOR

Techniques of Political Behavior
(*Mnemonic:* BIG CEO)

B Building coalitions—to have the alliance with right people
I Image building is creating positive impression reflected by **P**ersonality, **A**ppearance, and **S**tyle (PAS)
G Game playing-doing something insincere to gain political ends.
C *Controlling:* Information, Communication, and Agenda (ICA)
E Experts play politics—using outside experts
O *Others, according to STP:* Situations, Time, Pressure/Position/Place.

(In any organization, at any given moment, a number of people are seeking to gain and use power to achieve their own ends. This pursuit of power is political behavior. Ambiguous goals, scarce resources, changes in environment and technology, non-programmed decisions and organizational changes can influence political behavior.)

121. COMMUNICATION BARRIERS

Barriers to Effective Communication
(*Mnemonic:* SEMANTIC)

S Semantic/language barriers—due to differences in interpretations

E Emotion, strong feelings, emotions hinder effective communication
Environmental—heat, cold, poor ventilation affect communication

M Multi meaning words—perceptual barriers

A Any factor that interfaces with communication, e.g. Noise

N Network breakdown, Negative impact of fatigue

T Time constraints—message must be sent at proper time

I Information overload/inadequate

C Credibility/Confidentiality, Cultural barriers, Continuity gaps
Channel is inappropriate, Complex systems.

(Any breakdown in communication could be costly. The communication process may be interrupted by "noise" that is by anything that hinders communication. Communication is hindered by barriers and breakdowns the communication process. Recognizing these barriers and listening facilitate understanding.)

122. DISASTER PARADIGM CHECKLIST

(*Mnemonic:* DISASTER)

D Detection, Damage, Disruption

I Incident command

S Scene safety

A Assess hazards

S Support

T Triage/treatment

E Evacuation

R Recovery, Rescue.

123. PUBLIC EXPECTATIONS

Public Expectation from Medical Profession: **CARE**

C Care-cost of care, quality of care, preventive and promotive care

A Advice and attention

R Reassurance

E Education and expertise.

124. FREUD'S PERSONALITY THEORY

(Psychosexual Stages of Personality Development)

Sigmund Freud said, **GOPAL** Influenced Personality

(5 1 3 2 4)

G Genital stage (5) (Puberty on, sexual feelings toward others)

O Oral stage (1) (Birth to one year, mouth is associated with sexual pleasure)

P Phallic stage (3) (3–5 years, Focus of pleasure shifts to the genitals, "Oedipus Complex")

A Anal stage (2) (1–3 years, Anus is associated with pleasure, **Toilet** training can lead to fixation, if not handled correctly)

L Latent stage (4) (5—puberty, sexuality is dormant).

(Freud believed that these five key stages of childhood development influenced personality. Personality forms during the first few years of life, rooted in unresolved conflicts of early childhood. Strong conflict can fixate an individual at Stages 1, 2 or 3.)

125. QUALITY ACTIVITY

Three "P" for Quality Activity:

P1 *People:* Do the activities

P2 Processes, i.e. following instructions

P3 Paper work, documentation.

(Quality is never an accident, it is always the result of high intention, sincere effort, intelligent execution, and it represents the wise choice of many alternatives. In a truly competitive and global market, quality is the most important competitive strategy an organization can adopt.)

126. QUALITY MEASUREMENT

SOP Measures the Quality of Work

S *Structures:* Physical facilities

O *Outcome:* Final product, result

P *Process:* How the system works?

(Quality is a public issue and is vitally important in the field of hospital management. Quality in service sectors has to be ensured more by emphasis on processes rather than on final outcome. Monitoring and improving the process factors of care and quality management, therefore, assume importance as a means of regulating outcome of hospitalization. Quality management ensures improved outcome. Quality Improvement is the Science of Process Management. Healthcare delivery is a system made up of thousands of interlinked processes.)

127. SWOT ANALYSIS

What is SWOT Analysis?

S	*Strengths:*	What do we do well? (Indicators of environmental quality)
W	*Weaknesses:*	What is wrong not? (Indicators of environmental vulnerability)
O	*Opportunities:*	What possibilities exist? (Simulation of project to optimize the uses of the territory and to decrease environmental impacts)
T	*Threats:*	What can go wrong? (Quantitative evaluation of human impacts in territory).

(Strengths and Opportunities are ***helpful*** *to achieve objectives. Weakness and Threats are harmful to achieve objectives.)*

128. PUBLIC SPEAKING

ABC of Public Speaking

A Audience target

B Be prepared, Believe in what you say!

C Clarity and simplicity

D Dare to be speak

E End with acknowledgement and message

F Feedback is must.

129. CONFLICT AND CRISIS

In Situations of Crisis and Potential Conflict Always Remember: **STAR**

We need to:

S Stop
T Think
A Analyze
R Respond.

(Conflict is an inevitable part of life. Conflict may be intrapersonal, interpersonal or intergroup. Interpersonal conflicts are controllable and manager should not be bothered about them. Strategies applied to manage intergroup conflicts are avoiding the situation, diffusion and confrontation.)

130. LISTENER

Active Listeners should: SOLDER

S Squarely face the person, Stop talking first!
O Open posture adopt
L Lean slightly toward the other person
D Distance apart of about 1 meter, Distractions remove
E Eye contact maintain, Empathize with talker
R Relaxed.

(Listening is a key for understanding. It is a skill that can be developed by patience and practice.)

131. INTERVIEW

Objectives of the Interview: E4

E1 Engaging
E2 Empathizing
E3 Educating
E4 Enlisting.

(Interview is an important selection tool. It is an attempt to secure maximum amount of information from the candidate concerning his suitability for the job under consideration. It is a formal meeting to assess a job applicant.)

132. PREVENTION OF AIDS

ABCD of AIDS Prevention

A Abstinence till marriage
B Be faithful to one partner throughout life
C Condom use whenever necessary
D Discrimination against HIV positives and AIDS must stop.

(An ounce of prevention is better than ***pound of cure****, can be applied in case of AIDS, as there is no known cure for* ***AIDS*** *at present.)*

133. KARTAR SINGH COMMITTEE

Recommendations of Kartar Singh Committee:
(*Mnemonic:* MPW)

M Multipurpose workers (MPW) for delivery of health, family planning, and nutritional services to the rural areas are desirable
P Primary health center should serve 50,000 populations
W *Workers:* Male and female as health workers
(1 MHW/6–7 thousands pop, 1 FHW/10–12 thousands pop).

134. MASS TRIAGE

M Move
A Assess
S Sort
S Send.

[MASS triage is a disaster triage system that utilizes US military triage categories with a proven means of handling large numbers of casualties in a mass casualty incident (MCI).]

135. MEDICAL CONSULTATION

ABC of Medical Consultation

A Agree a management plans
B Build the relationship
C Collect data.

136. BREAKING BAD NEWS

Techniques for Breaking Bad News
(*Mnemonic:* SPIKES)

S Setting, sitting down, start with open questions
P Patient's perception—what patient thinks about his problems?
I *Invitation:* What he or she would like to know?
K Knowledge (giving medical facts)
E Explore emotions and empathizes
S Strategy and summary.

(Support system like social services, family, friends, etc. may involve in the strategy.)

137. DRUGS OF ABUSE

(*Mnemonic:* ALCOHOL)

A Alcohol, amphetamines
L LSD (Lysergic acid diethylamide)
C Cannabis, cocaine
O Opium
H Hypnotics, hallucinogens
O *Others:* Sedatives, phencyclidine
L Last but not least—inhalants.

(Any of these can cause an intoxication that may lead to delirium under some circumstances. Abuse of drugs and alcohol is one of the common social agents for disease causation.)

138. DELIRIUM

What causes Delirium?

(*Mnemonic:* WAIT AND WATCH)

W *Withdrawal:* Hypnotics, barbiturates
A *Acute metabolic:* Acid-base, electrolytes, liver/renal failure
I *Infections:* Meningitis, encephalitis, sepsis
T *Trauma:* Brain injury, burns
A Abuse of drugs
N Niacin deficiency, narcotics analgesics
D Deficiencies
W Worry about alcoholics
A *Acute vascular:* Shock, encephalopathy
T *Toxins/drugs*, too much or too little cortisol or glucose
C *CNS pathology:* SOL, stroke, seizures
H *Heavy metals:* Lead, manganese, mercury
Hypoxia can cause delirium.

(Delirium—a mental disturbance of relatively short duration usually reflecting a toxic state, marked by illusions, hallucinations, delusions, excitement, restlessness and incoherence.)

139. NATIONAL PROGRAMME FOR BLINDNESS CONTROL

Activities of National Programme for Control of Blindness

(*Mnemonic:* PROUDE)

P Provision of various ophthalmic services
R Recruitment of required ophthalmic manpower
O Outreaches activities and public awareness
U Upgradation of medical colleges and district hospitals
D Development of mobile eye units
E Establishment of regional institute of ophthalmology.

(Right to see is one of the basic human rights. To reduce the prevalence rate of blindness is a major objective of the programme. The program was launched in 1976 as 100% centrally sponsored program.)

140. NATIONAL HEALTH POLICY

Elements of National Health Policy (NHP)

(*Mnemonic:* MHP)

M1 Medical education
M2 Medical research
M3 Medical industry
M4 Management information system (MIS)
H1 Health education
H2 Health insurance and legislation
P1 Provision of PHC (primary healthcare)
P2 Practitioners of ISM (Indian System of Medicine)
P3 Population stabilizing
P4 Problems requiring urgent attention.

(The formulation of National Health Policy suggests major implications for restructuring of health services, reorientation and training of manpower, development of information system and periodic evaluation of healthcare services. Separate policies have been recommended on nutrition, population control, medical and health education. National Health Policy was evolved by the Government of India in 1983.)

141. CLASSIFICATION OF HOSPITALS

(*Mnemonic:* ABCDE)

A AYUSH Hospitals, according to ALS (average length of stay)
B *Based on Control/Ownership/Management:* Government and Non-Government (Profit and nonprofit)
Bed strength (200–500 beds)
(*Small hospital* <200 beds, *Medium Hospital:* 200–500 beds, *Large hospital* >500 beds)
C *Clinical basis:* General and special hospital
D Directory of Hospital listed different types of hospitals, such as SIR TG Hospital
E Expertise level (Primary Care/Secondary Care/Tertiary Care)

(Government Hospitals: Central/State/Local self/Public sector/under the act of legislation. Hospitals under various Ministries like Health, Home, Labor, and Defense as well as Railway Hospital are Central Government Hospital.)

142. PMR DEPARTMENT

PMR Department shall Require Space for Following Areas:
(*Mnemonic:* HOSPITAL)

H Hearing and speech therapy services
O OPD services, OT services, orthotic services, occupational therapy services
S Social and medical services
P Physiotherapy services, psychological and vocational services, prosthetic services, public utility services
I Indoor services
T Trolley and wheel chair services
A Administrative block and waiting area, attendants room
L Lift in vertical building.

(The department area should be barrier free with wide door, smooth, non-slippery flooring. Preferably the building should be single storied, if not possible, lift should be provided with wide door and back-up generator facility, in addition to the lifts, climbing ramp instead of stairs should be provided.)

143. COUNSELING

ABC of Counseling

A Assessing the staff's potentiality, attitude, stamina, etc.
B Building an index to helpful information
C Consulting sources of information, collect the data about counsellee
D Determining type of counseling required
E Evaluation of result
F Follow-up.

(Counseling is a process of helping a person to solve his problem by himself through advising and guiding. There are some basic counseling skills such as attending, observing, active-listening, summarizing, reflecting, questioning, silence, independence and concreting, etc. These skills are acquired by practice and experience. Good counseling helps the counsellee to develop the insight, also helps in establishing new goals and growth of confidence.)

144. NURSING SERVICES

Functions of Nursing Care Services:
(*Mnemonic:* OPQRST)

O Organization and administration of nursing services
P Provision of nursing care services, practice and education
Provision for financial resources
Procuring materials and supplies
Q Quality control
R Research in nursing care
S Supervision, system for data collection
Studies concerning all aspects of nursing services
Standards, objectives and policies formulation for nursing
T Training of nursing staff.

(A WHO Expert Committee on Nursing defines the Nursing Service as the part of the total health organization which aims to satisfy the nursing needs of the community. More than 75% of patients are merely satisfied by Nursing Services alone.)

145. PMR DEPARTMENT STAFF REQUIREMENT

Paramedical Manpower Requirement for PMR Department
(*Mnemonic:* PROSTHOTIC)

P Prosthetics, physiotherapist, psychiatrist
R Rehabilitation worker
O Occupational therapist
S Social worker
T Technician in various trades

H Hearing and speech therapist
O Orthotics
T Teacher
I Instructor, craft
C Counselor.

146. ALTERNATIVE SYSTEM OF MEDICINE
(*Mnemonic:* AYUSH)

AY Ayurvedic system of medicine
U Unani system of medicine
S Siddha system of medicine
H Homeopathic system of medicine.

147. INTELLIGENT BUILDING
Intelligent Building Possesses Power to TALK

T Think fast
A Anticipate the needs of owner, act fast.
L Learning ability
K Knowledge application.

(Besides beautiful, building should be intelligent and futuristic outlook too. Concept is catching up in the corporate buildings and will surely find its place in hospitals very soon as it can beneficially use all its capabilities.)

148. FULL FORM
What do these Stands for?
TR, AHU, RH, HEPA, BTU and HVAC?

AHU Air handling unit
BTU British thermal unit
HEPA High efficiency particulate air
HVAC Heating, ventilating and air-conditioning
RH Relative humidity
TR Tons refrigeration

(Ton means heat extraction capacity of AC plant.
One ton = heat extraction rate (HER) of 12,000 BTU per hour
One TR unit can suffice for a room up to 12 sq. meter.)

149. VED-VEIN ANALYSIS

It is used to Classify the Intrinsic Value of a Spare and is Explained as:

VED Vital, essential, desirable

VEIN Vital, essential, important, normal

Vital: Nonavailability will cause considerable loss (top management control it)

Essential: Nonavailability cause moderate loss (middle management control it)

Desirable: Nonavailability will cause minor loss (lower management control it).

(VED analysis is based on critical values and shortage cost of items and is depend on objectives of the hospital.)

150. STORAGE AND PRESERVATION

Storage and Preservation Remember D10:

D1 Documented and correctly inventoried
D2 Duly protected from ill effects of weather
D3 Dirt, dust and damage protection
D4 Dampness, guarded against it
D5 Direct sunlight avoided
D6 Dryness, guarded against it
D7 Dust free air-conditioning storage
D8 Dry room for electrodes
D9 Delicately preservation for expensive spares in their original packing
D10 Dehydrated silica gel should be used.

151. ENGINEERING SERVICE DEPARTMENT

Functional Areas of Engineering Service Department:
(*Mnemonic:* A to G)

A Air conditioning and refrigeration services management
B *Biomedical equipment:* Maintenance and repair
C *Civil assets:* Maintenance and repair
D Department wise miscellaneous items
Department deals with water supply and sewage system
E Electrical power provisioning
Equipment, instruments, vehicles: Maintenance and repair
F Fire detection and protection system
G General safety and security system.

(Engineering service is a lifeline of the hospital, hence planning of engineering services has to be based on zero-failure concept. Engineering hazards are mainly due to faulty planning and unsoundness of structures to withstand natural calamities and manmade disasters.)

152. FIRE SAFETY

ABC Fire Safety in the Hospital:

A Alarm system as per National Building Code guideline
B Building coming under Group C-1 (Industrial)
C Containment of fire
D Detection of fire is ultimate aim in design
Design and select high rating structural members
E Emergency exit is one of the prime requirements
F Fire protected and smoke free escape routes
Fire rating of 2–4 hours depending on occupancy
Fire walls to limit fire spread.

(No safety program is complete without training and awareness.)

153. WELL BEING

Essential Minimum Requirements of Well-being
(*Mnemonic:* NEWS)

N Nutrition
E Education
W Water
S Shelter.

(WHO definition of health introduces the concept of well-being. It has two components: Subjective and Objective. Subjective component of well-being is referred to as "quality of life". Objective component of well-being is referred to as "standard of living".)

154. EPIDEMIC FORECASTING

Techniques of Epidemic Forecasting Tabulation of Data on "**AIDS**" for at Least Three Years (monthly and yearly basis)

A Age group
I Incidence/prevalence rate of the disease
D Disease
S Sex-wise incidence and prevalence.

(The major techniques of epidemics forecasting is based on trend analysis of particular disease over a period of time. Comparison of data for seasonal and cyclic variation. Plotting different graphs and preparing spot maps ***to detect*** *regional variations.)*

155. ELECTRIC SUPPLY FAILURE

Main Causes of Failure of Electric Supply are:
(*Mnemonic:* C1, C2, C3, C4, C5)

C1 Circuit at fault (short circuit)
C2 Carelessness during lying of cables
C3 Cables deforming insulation due to physical pressure
C4 Crimping, abrasion due to mechanical damage
C5 Cable sheath moistened due to any reasons.

156. WALKING AROUND INSPECTION

Three Senses Inspection Points:
(*Mnemonic:* HOT)

H *Hear:* Unusual noise

(Air, steam or gas leak-hissing, banging—doors or windows not secured, barking-dogs on the premises, chirping—bird's nests, dripping-fluid leaks, grinding—lack of maintenance, silence, humming—machinery not working properly)

O Observe or seeing

(Air, lubricant leakage, broken glass panes, corrosion, discoloration, deterioration, electric sparks, fluid leakage, garbage and refuse collection)

T Touch or feel

(Airleaks from ducts-breeze, cold-no hot water or steam flow, draught-open doors, broken windows, shaking, and vibration-machine out of balance, hot-bearing, shafts).

(There are five senses, optimum use of them one can develop sixth sense, common sense which is not so common is seventh sense, last one is non-sense that is notorious too!.)

157. SERVICE MARKETING MIX

Seven "P" for Services Marketing Mix:

P1 People
P2 Process
P3 Product
P4 Price
P5 Place
P6 Promotion
P7 Physical evidence.

(Service marketing requires a different treatment as compared to goods marketing because of distinctive characteristics of services. These include intangibility, heterogeneity, inseparability of production, consumption and

perishability. Because of these characteristics, the traditional 4P marketing mix is inadequate and service marketing entails an extended 7P marketing mix for services.)

158. FLOW OF GOODS

Generally use Methods are as follows:

(*Mnemonic:* FALSE)

F *FIFO method:* "First in, first out" method is mostly use.
(The oldest cost should be charged)

A Average cost method, average cost of each item should be charged

L *LIFO method:* "Last in, first out"—most current cost should be charged.

S *Specific cost method*—The most realistic valuation of ending inventory as well as flow of costs. It is suitable for physical verification of inventories made round the year.

E Else.

(Flow of goods is directly related to flow of costs, flow of costs depends upon the method used, which are listed above.)

159. EQUIPMENT SELECTION

Steps for Equipment Selection:

(*Mnemonic:* SCIENTIFIC)

S Stick to specification not the brand
Supplier selection and purchase procedure

C Coefficient is applied to assess equipment utilization

I Installation on turn-key basis

E Economically consideration like cost, consumables, contract, etc.

N Need assessment, justifying the need of particular equipment

T Training of staff to handle the equipment efficiently

I Insurance and freight are covered up to nearest port with customer clearance facility.

F Forward booking in fluctuating foreign exchange
Facility for back-up power supply should be considered.

I Installation engineer should involve in site selection/preparation

C Cost consciousness and warranty with spares

Continuous supply of consumables

Contract for maintenance and after sale service must be considered.

160. TYPES OF INVENTORY CONTROL

Types of control	*Basis*	*Main use*
1. ABC (Always better control)	Value of consumption of item	Control inventory value
2. VED (Vital, essential, desirable)	Criticality of item	Inventory control of spares
3. FSN (Fast, slow, non-moving)	Consumption pattern of items	Control obsolescence
4. GOLF (Government ordinary, local, foreign)	Source of supply	Procurement strategies
5. HML (High, medium, low)	Unit price of items	Control purchase
6. SDE (Scarce, difficult, easy to obtain)	Problems of procurement	Lead time analysis and purchasing strategies
7. SOS (Seasonal, of seasonal)	Nature of supply	Procurement and holding strategies for seasonal items
8. XYZ	Value of items in store	Review inventories

(Inventory classification is must for better management of inventory. Classification of inventory is based on Pareto's Law. While studying the economic pattern of a given city, Pareto, a German Economist found that 20% of the people have got 80% of the total money and rest of the 80% of the people were having 20% of the money.)

161. HERZBERG'S HYGIENE FACTORS

(*Mnemonic:* POWERS)

P Personal life
O Organizational policy and administration
W Working conditions
E Expert supervision (technical)
R Relations (interpersonal) with head and colleagues
S Salary, status, security (3S).

(Hygiene needs are related to the physical and psychological context of the work—comfortable work environment, pay, job security. Unsatisfied hygiene needs create dissatisfaction; satisfaction of hygiene needs does not lead to motivation or job satisfaction.)

162. CENTRALIZATION VERSUS DECENTRALIZATION

IDEA of Centralization versus Decentralization

(*Mnemonic:* IDEA: Institution, decision making, everything, authority)

	Centralization	***Decentralization***
Institution	Small	Medium and large
Decision making	By higher authority, not at workplace	By responsible person for job, at work place
Everything	Which goes to reduce it?	Which goes to increase it?
Authority	Systemic reservation of authority	Systemic delegation of authority at central

163. MECHANIZED LAUNDRY: EQUIPMENT REQUIREMENT

Equipment Requirement for the Mechanized Laundry are:

(*Mnemonic:* STEAM BED)

S Steam bed press, scale, weighing
T Trolleys
Tables for ironing
E Electric iron, extractor-hydro
A Air compressor

M *Machines:* Washing, sluice, sewing, calendaring
B Boilers
E Extinguisher—fire
D Driers.

164. QUALITY IN HOUSEKEEPING SERVICE

Indicators of Quality in Housekeeping Services
(*Mnemonic:* AIDS)

A *Automation:* Degree
I Incinerator availability
D *Disinfectants:* Its effectiveness checks or not
S *Staff:* Total number, training, team spirit.

165. CENTRAL SECURITY CONTROL ROOM

5M for Central Security Control Room

M1 Monitor security of sensitive areas
M2 MIS report for management on security aspects
M3 Mobile patrolling all the time
M4 Monitor performance of security staff
M5 Movement of man, material and motor vehicles—keep computerized records.

166. AMBULANCE

Criteria to call a vehicle as an ambulance

An Ambulance should be
Built to
Cope with emergency
Designed
Equipped and staffed in that ways.

(Ambulance was first used in France, in 1762. Objective of ambulance service is to provide prompt emergency treatment, safe transportation with continued treatment to hospital for further treatment.)

167. LABORATORY HAZARDS

'HIS': Laboratory Hazards

H *Handling:* Infectious materials and broken glassware
I *Inhalation:* Inoculation and poisonous fumes
Inflammable chemicals and gas leakages
S *Swallowing materials:* Infectious and corrosive.

(Caution: Avoid mouth pipetting as far as possible.)

3S for Safety Precautions in the Laboratory

S1 **Safe** laboratory procedure
S2 **Standard** (basic) of laboratory design, operation and equipment
S3 **Selection** and use of biosafety equipment.

168. FULL FORM

Elaborate the Terms

LASER, RPAD, BRIT, BARC, DRP, RPSD

BARC **B**habha **A**tomic **R**esearch **C**entre
BRIT **B**oard of **R**adiation **I**sotope **T**echnology
DRP **D**ivision of **R**adiological **P**rotection
LASER **L**ight **A**mplification by **S**timulated **E**mission of **R**adiation
RPAD **R**adiological **P**hysics and **A**dvisory **D**ivision
RPSD **R**adiation **P**rotection **S**ervice **D**ivision.

169. HEALTH SERVICES

4I for Health Services

I1 **Inconsistency**
(Both the composition and quality of health services used vary from person to person and from event to event)
I2 **Intangibility**
(Consumer cannot see, smell, taste, feel or hear a medical service)
I3 **Inseparability**
(Production and consumption take place simultaneously)

14 Inventory

(Most medical services cannot be stockpiled).

170. FIXED COST
IRDA is a CASE of Fixed Costs

I Insurance
R Rent, repairs and maintenance
D Depreciation
A Administrative expenses

Fixed costs are:

Constant costs, irrespective of the changes in the volume
At any cost, it cannot be avoided
Same costs whether the production is zero
Essential cost for the business.

171. WRITING SKILL
Valuable Writing 'TIPS'

T Topic sentence
To the point, clear, concise
I Inverted pyramid, illustrations and examples use
P Plain english, personal pronouns whenever applicable
S Short and simple sentences/words.

(A clearly written message helps to avoid semantic and physical barriers. It reduces the possibilities of misunderstanding and misinterpretation. The word becomes powerful once it is written.)

172. QUALITY OF MESSAGE
Quality of Message Content
(*Mnemonic:* C1, C2, C3, C4, C5 and C6)

C1 Correctness
C2 Completeness
C3 Clarity

C4 **C**oncreteness
C5 **C**ourtesy
C6 **C**onciseness.

173. LISTENING SKILL

ABC of Listening Skill
(LISTENING: THE ART of COMMUNICATION)

A **A**nalyze the message
B **B**egin with an open mind
C **C**oncentrate and catch up the key words
D **D**etermine the speaker's approach to messages
E **E**ye contact with the speaker
F **F**eedback is must
G **G**ive the judgment after entire message has heard.

(Listening is not so easy but one should cultivate the art of good listening for effective communication. Good listening skill helps to concentrate properly. Lack of listening acts as an obstacle in the way of communication.)

174. RELATIONSHIP

3C for a Successful Relationship

C1 **C**ommunication
C2 **C**ommunication
C3 **C**ommunication.

(Effective communication is the foundation of relationship. It is impossible to have a human relation without communication and vice versa.
We have to remember:
Much communication is unconscious
Much communication is unintentional
Much communication is incongruent.)

175. STANDARDS OF MEDICAL CARE

Five Intra-mural Factors for Deterioration of Standards of Medical Care

(*Mnemonic:* TPR BP)

T *Training:* Inadequate training to the staff

P ***Policies***: Inadequate

R *Rules and regulation:* Inadequate

Resources: Inadequate and underutilized

B **B**udgetary planning and control is very poor

P **P**rocedures are not proper.

176. RIGHTS OF THE PATIENT

'SPECIAL' Rights of the Patient

S *Safety:* Right to safety

P *Privacy:* Right to privacy

E *Education:* Right to education/know

C There are seven 'C'

- **C1** *Choose:* Right to choose and to be heard
- **C2** *Confidentiality:* Right to confidentiality
- **C3** *Communication:* Right to communication
- **C4** *Consent:* Right to consent
- **C5** *Consultation:* Right to consultation
- **C6** Continuity of care
- **C7** *Complains:* Right to complains

I *Information:* Right to information (RTI)

A *Access:* Right to access to care

L Last but not least at least, respect and dignity to the patient.

(Health is a fundamental human right. Patient rights are developed on the notion of human right, depending on sociocultural norms. Patient rights vary according to countries and jurisdictions.)

177. ORGANIZATION

'CORE' Characteristics of an Organization

C *Communication:* Lifeline of the organization
O *Objectives:* Without it, no reason to exist
R Rules and regulation
E Efforts.

(An organization is a mechanism with which a management directs controls and co-ordinates the activities of man. An organization is a machine of management in its achievement of the ends determined by its administration.)

178. UNSAFE BEHAVIOR

ABC Analysis of Unsafe Behavior

A **A**ntecedent—Event that triggers a behavior
B **B**ehavior—Observable action (measurable)
C **C**onsequence—Outcome or result of behavior.

179. HUMAN RELATION PROBLEMS

Be "SOFT" to Solve Human Relation Problems

S **S**eparate fact from ISO (imagination, sentiment, opinion)
O **O**pen minded
F **F**riendly discussion
T **T**emper control.

(Remember: If you let off a man at any point, assure him when you will take action and be prepared to keep the promise you make.)

180. PERSONNEL MANAGER

Functions of a Personnel Manager:
(*Mnemonic:* POSD RBC)

P Planning
O Organizing

S Staffing
D Directing
R Reporting
B Budgeting
C Coordinating the work of those who are entrusted with the performance of operative functions.

181. HUMAN RESOURCE ACTION PROGRAMS

(*Mnemonic:* CALL THEM)

C Communication participation
A Administration of wage and salary
L Labor relations
L Loss and profits to the employee
T Training and development
H Human resource forecasting and planning
E Employment and related acts
Evaluation techniques
M Management development programs.

182. HOSPITAL ORGANIZATION

(Uniqueness of the Hospital Organization)

Hospital is a "SPECIAL" Organization, which differs from other organizations in certain distinct ways:

S Service organization, no clear conceptualization of output
P Personalized service specific to each individual patient's need
E Ethical norms area must for the hospitals
Emergency care is extended, irrespective of patient's condition, caste, costs, or contagious status.
C Code of behavior is expected of all the staff
Confidentiality should be preserved all the time
I Indiscipline has no room in the hospital
In spite of an individual hospital's objectives, hospitals are becoming increasingly responsive to health needs of surrounding community.

A Areas that cannot be categorized as purely clinical/administrative
L Long-lasting operations in spite of certain work constraints
Last but not least, Litigation of laws is always there.

183. GROUPS OF HOSPITAL SERVICES

Distinct Groups of Hospital Services

(*Mnemonic:* A to G)

A Ancillary services
B Business, utility services and specialized services
C Clinical services
D Diagnostic services
E Emergency services
F Fiscal services (Finance, internal audit, stores, cash, computers and hospital information system (HIS), administration, legal and labor services)
G General services (teaching/training).

184. INTERNAL CONTROL

"REAL" Internal Control

R Revenue (pt. revenue, account receivable, grants, donations)
E Expenditure (salary, supplies and expenses, repair and maintenance)
A Assets (land and building, cash investment, inventory, equipment)
L Liabilities (loan, accounts payable, specific purpose fund).

(It is mandatory for the administrator to have a control over the finances of the hospital. Administrator must be conversant with what is financial status of the hospital. Adequate accounting system should be instituted.)

185. CONSUMER FORUM

Consumer Dispute Redressal Agencies

(*Mnemonic:* CPA)

C Complaints and compensation
Complaints where compensation claimed <₹ 5 lacs (District)
Complaints where compensation claimed >5 lacs, <20 lacs (State)
Complaints and compensation claimed >₹ 20 lacs (National)

P *President:* District judge at District forum
High Court judge at State commission
Supreme Court judge at National commission

Persons: Two persons known for ability, integrity, knowledge of economics, law, commerce, accounting, industry or administration, one of whom shall be a woman, District and State Commission consisting of three persons, National Commission has five persons.

A An Appeal
Appeal against the order of District Forum lies with the State Commission within 30 days.
Appeal against the order of the State Commission lies with the National Commission within 30 days.
Appeal against the order of the National Commission lies with the Supreme Court within 30 days.

(The Consumer Protection Act was passed by the Parliament in 1986 with a view to provide for the better protection of the interest of the consumers for settlement of consumer disputes; under the Section (9), the Act provides for the constitution of the ***Consumer Forum****. Under the Act, a Consumer needs not to pay any fees. Dispute is required to be decided in three months, if it does not involve examination by an expert or adducing expert evidence.)*

186. NEGLIGENCE'S REMEDY

"LIC" is a Legal Remedy when Negligence

L *Law of tort:* Breach of contract, whether patient pays or not
I Indian Medical Council Act, 1956
C *Criminal liability:* IPC Section 304A
Civil liability: Indian Contract Act-sections 73 and 74
Consumer Protection Act, 1986.

(Negligence is a careless act and may result in harm. A person is said to be negligent when he/she acts without due care in regard to the harmful consequences of his/her action.)

187. HOSPITAL COST

Factors Affecting Hospital Costs

(*Mnemonic:* MEDICAL COST)

M Medical practice style, moral and motivation of staff
E Efficient management system
D Drug of choice
I Input versus output
C Complex cases raise the cost per patient
A Activity levels, average length of stay
L Larger the volume of services, lower the average cost
C Competition between hospitals
O *Occupancy level:* High occupancy leads to lower average cost
S Service quality (quality is not costly)
T Technologies are usually expensive
Training and education programs.

188. COST CONTAINMENT

"REST" to the Staff to Reduce Cost in Hospital

R Rationalization of staffing patterns
E Education about costing of services
S Standards and norms of staffing based on work studies
T Training and motivate to all to contain cost.

(In health care, the best way to contain costs is to improve quality and motivate the staff.)

189. HOSPITAL EXPENDITURE

"CASHIER" Affecting Hospital Expenditure!

C Cost containment approach, cost consciousness, cost-effectiveness,
Cost awareness, cost monitoring, cost management to contain costs
Competition between hospitals result in higher costs
Computerization of accounting and administrative records

A *Activity level:* Higher the patient turnover, lower the unit cost
Approach like camp, day-care surgery, and quality management

S Service intensity, Specialization leads to higher cost/patient day,
Shutting down electricity when not required reduces cost
Service contract and privatization of underutilized services

H Hospital size and design affecting the expenditures

I *Investment:* Availability of costly equipments and facilities lead to higher cost to the patient
Instituting the department-wise quarterly budgets, information booklets, introduction to multi-skilled staff, reduces costs

E Eliminating wastage and pilferage
Efficient management system reduces costs

R *Reimbursement pattern:* Payment by third parties increases cost.

190. WARD RECORDS

Documents and Records to be Maintained in the Ward
(*Mnemonic:* IT CASE CARD)

I Instructions book which the nurses carried with her
Indent books for various stores like medical stores, instruments, linen, and dispensary

T Telephone message book

C Case cards, complaints book for repair and maintenance

A Admission registers

S Stock register for FILE (Furniture, Instruments, Linen, Equipment)

E ESR and weight records for TB patients

C *Charts:* Total peripheral resistance blood pressure (TPRBP), input/output (I/O), etc.

A Attendance book for medical officer (MO) in case of emergency calls

R Records of laboratory, radiology and weight

D Discharge register

S Suggestion book.

191. INDUCTION PROGRAM

Contents of Induction Program

(*Mnemonic:* WHO IS GPSC TOP)

W Wage and salary description
H Holidays and leave details
O Overtime criteria
I Institution: History, aims and objectives
Introduction to all supervisors
S Safety measures
G Grievance procedure
P Personnel policies and name of key personnel
S Standing orders and disciplinary procedure
C Clear concept of job
T Training, transfer policies
Terms and conditions of services
O Opportunity for promotions
P Personnel benefits and services.

192. INTERNATIONAL BUYING

Problems of International Buying

(*Mnemonic:* PROBLEM OF CUSTOM)

P Problems in custom clearance, political uncertainties
Problems in insurance claims settlement
R Restricted shipping and cargo-carrying capacity
Rackets in imports leading to international maritime frauds
O Outflow of precious limited foreign exchange
B Buyer can pretend the quality of imported items with a manufacture's guarantee certificate
L Long lead time
Legal system at international level leading to many difficulties
E Experience and technical skills are a must
M Maintenance and repair contract costly rather than impossible

O Open discussion with foreign supplier regarding price, quality and contract is a must

F Fluctuating foreign currency
Flash strike on minor differences in major port such as Kolkata, Mumbai.

C Communication difficulties
Congested port facilities
Cope with clumsy commercial practices and commodity specification

U Unreliable delivery schedules

S Screw-driver technology is harmful

T Transportation charges are very high
Threats of terrorism

O *Others:* Government's policies/license lengthy procedure

M Money devaluation and global inflationary trends.

193. EMOTIONAL CONTROL

Essential Steps to Emotional Control
(*Mnemonic:* A1, A2, A3, A4, and A5)

A1 *Awareness:* Means being aware of the emergence of the subtlest of emotions.

A2 *Acknowledge:* Means taking responsibility for the emotion by understanding and acknowledging that I am the creator of the emotion, not someone or something else.

A3 *Acceptance:* Fully accept the emotion without resisting it.

A4 *Ascend:* This is the moment of full detachment from both the emotion and the inner source of emotion. In the process of detached observation, the emotion is losing its power. And it is only through detached observation that the emotion will begin to dissipate and eventually dissolve.

A5 *Attune:* Means returning our attention to the very center of ourselves where our inner peace and power are to be found.

(Emotion means strong feelings, such as love, sorrow, anger, fear, joy, sadness, acceptance, disgust, expectancy, surprise, etc. Emotion is one of the major communication barriers. Don't be emotional, control it through above steps.)

194. EQUIPMENT INFORMATION

Each Equipment has "AYURVEDIC" Information

A Asset title
Y Year of acquisition/purchased
U Useful life
R Replacement cost
V Various cost centers to which initially assigned
E Each equipment should bear all these details
D Date of capital improvements
I Inflation rate since purchased
C Cost of capital improvements.

195. MANAGER'S MORAL

5R's as Moral Principles for Managers

R1 *Role and responsibility:* Judge by their consequences
R2 *Results:* Achieve the greatest results for maximum people
R3 *Right and respect:* Basic human rights should be respected
R4 Rules for everyone without bias
R5 Rewards should be administered impartially, fairly, equitably.

196. PRINCIPLES OF ORGANIZATION

(*Mnemonic:* SCALAR)

S Scalar chain
Span of control
Specialization
Simplicity
C Co-ordination, Continuity
Command
A Authority, Adaptability
Aims/Objectives
L Labor division
A Arrangement of administrative function
R Responsibility

197. INTENSIVE CARE UNIT: A TO Z

A Airway management, ambu bag, aspect of care
B Blood pressure, bed sore, breathing monitoring
C Consciousness level, circulation, cough reflex, catheter care
D Drains, delivery of drugs, dressing, doctor visit, documentation
E ECG, Environment, Equipment for therapeutic and monitoring
F Fluid status, facilities and fixtures
G Gag reflex, GI losses
H Head positioning, Heart rate
I Insensible losses, IV line, IVF, ICCU
J Jugular venous pulse, Justice-distributive
K Kindness, Know why?
L Labeling, Limbs care, Liaison with parent unit
M Mouth care, Monitoring-close, Medication
N Nutrition, Nociception, Nursing care, Nourishing areas
O Observation, Oxygenation, Orientation, Orders follow up
P Pulse, Peristalsis, Physiotherapy, Punctuality
Q Quiet surroundings, Quality assessment
R Respiratory rate, Restraint, Reporting, Responsibility
S Suctioning, Stress ulcer, Sepsis screening
T Temperature chart, Timely intervention
U Urine output, Unambiguous protocol
V Ventilator, Visitors in waiting zone
W Wound care, Weight, Watch
X Xerosis
Y Yield management, why?
Z Zestful care to the critical patient.

(ICUs were developed to concentrate three critical components—the seriously sick patients, highly skilled staff with knowledge and experience to treat the patient and to use equipment for better results at reduced costs.)

198. DIMENSION OF QUALITY

(*Mnemonic:* RATE)

R *Reliability:* Accuracy
Responsiveness
A *Assurance:* To inspire trust and confidence
T *Tangibility:* Visible evidence
E *Empathy:* Feeling difficulties for others
Reserved: Poor communicator, insensitive to morale issues.

199. ORGANIZATIONAL EFFECTIVENESS

Components of Organizational Effectiveness
(*Mnemonic:* GET monitoring system)

G Good management—developed by good leadership
E Effective strategy—developed by effective leadership
T Team members should be talented and motivated
M Monitoring systems to keep track of the above.

(Effectiveness is the degree to which organization realizes its goals. Effectiveness does not guarantee efficiency and vice versa. Organizational effectiveness can be measured by goal approach, functional approach and system-resource approach.)

200. CYCLE OF THE FIVE D's

D1 DO...When you can
D2 DELEGATE...When you can't do
D3 DELAY...When you can't delegate
D4 DELETE...When you can't delay
D5 DO...When you can't delete.

201. PERSONALITY TRAITS

"A CEO" is for Major Five Personality Traits

A Agreeableness (Soft-hearted/Suspicious/Ruthless/Trusting)
C Conscientiousness (Organized/Disorganized/Careful/Careless)

E Extraversion (Sociable/Sober/Talkative/Assertive)
Emotional stability (Secure/Anxiety/Nervous/Tense/Calm)
O Openness (Practical/Imaginative/Independent/Conforming).

(Five personality traits have recently emerged from research as being especially related to job performance. The identification of the above five traits that relate to performance indicate the important role that personality plays in organizational behavior.)

202. FREUD'S PERSONALITY THEORY (MRP)

M *Morality (Superego):* Our urge to do "what is right".
Conscious, Preconscious, Unconscious
R *Reality (Ego):* Balance between Superego and Id
Secondary process thinking, Preconscious
P *Pleasure (Id):* Our primitive instinct,
Primary process thinking, Unconscious.

203. MEETINGS
Preparing for a Meeting
(*Mnemonic:* PROGRAME)

P Power
R Resources
O Other consequences
G *Goal:* Define goals
R Relationship and history
A Alternatives?, Agenda
M Minutes for meeting, Meeting preparation
E Expected outcomes.

(Meeting is an organized gathering for a discussion. Meetings generally work through a planned agenda.)

204. HOSPITAL DEPARTMENTS

(*Mnemonic:* A to G)

A Administrative zone
Ambulatory zone
B Board of the hospital (Governing body)
C Critical zone (OT/LR)
D Diagnostic zone
E Entrance zone (Reception/Registration/Record storage)
F Facility zone (Kitchen/CSSD/Laundry)
G General/special ward.

205. ICU DIRECTOR

Role of Director of ICU

(*Mnemonic:* CARE)

C Continuity clinical care provider
A Authority and administrative matter act as spokesman
R Responsible for purchasing and functioning of equipment
Review all treatment regimens with staff
Research activities
E Education and supervision of junior staff.

(Besides clinical duties, ICU Director has above all responsibilities. Each ICU must have a Director in the best interest of the patients. Consult parent unit, in case of outline of treatment.)

206. QUALITY HEALTH CARE

Components of Quality Health Care

(*Mnemonic:* STEP)

S Safety first
T Time is essence
E E3: Equitable, Effective and Efficient
P Patient centered

(Quality of care is the degree to which health services for individuals and populations increase the likelihood of desired health outcomes and are consistent with the current professional knowledge. Providing high quality of care with a maximum of safety for the patient within an affordable and balanced budget—is a challenge for every hospital management.)

207. TIME WASTERS

Major Time Wasters

(*Mnemonic:* PLAN)

P Procrastination
Problems with priorities

L Low self-esteem

A Afraid to delegate

N NO: Not want to say "NO".

(Time: Non-renewable Resource
Once it is gone, it is gone. You will never see this moment again.
Do not waste time in unnecessary arguments, even if you win, you lose in goodwill.
A man who dares to waste one hour of time has not discovered the value of life.)

208. PROBLEM SOLVING

(*Mnemonic:* SLATE)

S State the problem

L Look for areas of agreement

A Alternatives exploration

T Try a solution

E Evaluate results.

(The difference between what we do and what we are capable of doing would suffice to solve most of the world's problems.)

209. PRICE

Base of Price Charges

(*Mnemonic:* RATE)

R Resources consumed

A Admission charge

T Time basis

E Element of treatment/services.

210. HOUSEKEEPING SERVICES

Key Responsibilities of the Housekeeping Services

(*Mnemonic:* CADRE)

C Cleanliness to all

A Attain and maintain clean housekeeping equipment

D Disposal of hospital waste

R Replace supplies in utility room

E Exterminate bugs and pets.

211. MORTUARY EQUIPMENT

(*Mnemonic:* ABCDEFGH)

A Autopsy table

B Baw and meat-cutting saw

C Cold chamber, chromatography kits

D Doctors' room with table, chairs and telephone

E Equipment such as large sinks, spectrophotometer, sterilizer, weighing scale, X-ray

F Fume chamber

G Glass cupboard

H High pressure liquid chromatography.

212. RADIATION SAFETY

Radiation Safety Monitoring Practices

All persons who work with ionizing radiation must wear "BAG"

B *Badge:* A small film badge to record the dosage received during their work

A *Apron:* Routine use of radiation-proof apron

G *Gloves:* Protective gloves must be worn by a person who will be in the X-ray beam during exposure.

Management by Definitions (MBD)

Management is a broad term. There are many explanations on this term. Besides business concern, management is essential for all type of enterprises. Every organization has objectives of its own which can be achieved with cooperative efforts of several personnel through the process of management. At least two persons are essential to form a management. Management is an activity of a man who struggles for better living in the complex and competitive world. In this global scenario, management meets the challenge of change. There are eight M's in the business. These are men, money, materials, machines, methods, motivation, market, and management. Without management, all are remaining merely as resources. Management is top most of all other M's. Management has control over other remaining M's. Management means:

1. Management is commonly defined as "getting work done through other people".
2. Management can be defined as the art of bringing together available resources including the abilities of different people and organizing them in scientific and orderly manner, to achieve the desired goals of the organization.
3. Management is the process of designing and maintaining an environment in which individuals, working together in groups, to accomplish selected aims efficiently.
4. Management is the process undertaken by one or more persons to coordinate the activities of the other persons, to achieve results not attainable by any one person acting alone.
5. Management is a process of planning, organizing, directing and controlling the activities of others to obtain organizational objectives.
6. Management is the power to determine what shall happen to the personalities and happiness of entire people, the power to shape the destiny of a nation and of all the nations which make up the world (E Demock).
7. Management is the art of getting things done by a group of people with the effective utilization of available resources.
8. Management is an organ; organs can be described and defined only through their functions (Peter Drucker).
9. Management is not people; it is an activity like walking, reading, swimming or running. People who perform management can be designated as managers (Terry).

10. Management is the function of executive leadership anywhere (Ralph C Davis).
11. Management is concerned with seeing that the job gets done, its tasks all center on planning and guiding the operations that are going in the enterprise (EFL Brech).
12. Management is what a manager does (Allan Louis).
13. Management is defined for conceptual, theoretical and analytical purpose as that process by which managers create, direct maintain and operate purposive organization through systemic, coordinated cooperative human effort (Mc Farland).
14. To manage is to forecast and plan, to organize, to compound, to co-ordinate and to control (Henry Fayol).
15. Management is the art of getting things done through and with an informally organized group (Harold Koontz).
16. Management is that function of an enterprise which concerns itself with direction and control of various activities to attain business objectives. It is essentially an executive function; it deals with the active direction of the human effort (William Spriegel).
17. Management is the process by which a cooperative group directs actions towards common goals (Joseph L Massie).
18. Management is a technique by means of which the purposes and objectives of a particular human group are determined, clarified and effectuated (Elmore Peterson and EG Plowman).
19. Management is the process of getting things done through the agency of a community. The functions of management are the handling of a community with a view to fulfilling the purposes for which it exists (Sir Charles Reynold).
20. Management embraces all duties and functions that pertain to the initiation of an enterprise, its financing, the establishment of all major policies, the provision of all necessary equipment, the outlining of the general form of organization under which the enterprise is to operate and the selection of the principal officers (Kimball and Kimball).
21. Good management or scientific management achieves a social objective with the best use of human and material energy and time and with satisfaction for the participants and the public (Mary Cushing Niles).
22. Management consists of getting things done through others. Manager is one who accomplishes the objectives by directing the efforts of others (S George).

23. Management is the art of inspiring and directing the people (James D Mooney and Alan C Railey).
24. Management is the art of knowing what you want to do and then seeing that it is done in the best and cheapest way (FW Taylor).
25. Management is the art of getting things done through the efforts of other people (Lawrence A Appleby)
26. Management is the art of securing maximum results with a minimum effort so as to secure maximum prosperity for the employer and employee and give the public the best possible services (John F Mee).
27. The art of getting things done through other people (AMA).
28. The organization and control of human activity are directed towards specific ends (RM Currie).
29. Management is the creation and maintenance of an internal environment in an enterprise where individuals, working in groups, can perform efficiently and effectively towards the attainment of group's goals. It is the art of getting the work done through and with people in formally organized groups (Knootz and O'Donnell).
30. Management is the force that integrates men and physical plant into an effective operating unit (Keith and Gubellini).
31. The job of management is to make cooperative endeavor to function properly. A manager is one who gets things done by working with the people and other resources in order to reach an objective (Newman, Summer and Warren).
32. Management is the force which leads, guides and directs an organization in the accomplishment of a predetermined object (JN Schulze).
32. Management proper is the function in industry concerned in the execution of policy, within the limits set up by the administration and the employment of the organization for the particular objectives set before it (Oliver Sheldon).
33. Management is centered in the administrators or managers of the firm who integrate men, material and money into an effective operating limit (Wheeler).
34. Management is the principally a task of planning, coordinating, motivating and controlling the effort of others towards a specific objective (Dr James Lundy).
35. Management is the process and the agency through which the execution of policy is planned and supervised (GE Milward).
36. Management is the process and agency which directs and guides the operations of an organization in the realizing of established aims (Ordway Tead).

37. Management is the group of activities, which draft plans, prepares policies and arranges men, money, machine and materials required to achieve the objectives.
38. Management is the activity of a man who struggles for better living in the complex and competitive world.
39. Management is the process consisting of the functions of planning, organizing, staffing, directing and controlling the operations to achieve specified objectives.
40. Management is the practice of continually and consciously shaping organization.
41. Management is an art of getting things done through people.
42. Management means more than just—what is happening inside a particular organization.
43. Management is the process of reaching organizational goals by working with and through people and other resources.
44. Management is the process, composed of a set of interrelated social and technical functions and activities, occurring within a formal organizational setting for the purpose of accomplishing predetermined objectives through utilization of human and other resources.
45. Management is the process by which an organization employs its resources (Men, Money, Material, and Machine) to achieve predetermined objectives.
46. Management is a multi-purpose organ which has three jobs, two of which are directly related to personnel managing a business: managing managers and managing workers and the works.
47. Management is the accomplishment of results through the efforts of other people (Lawrence Appley).
48. Management may be thought of as the process of allocating an organization's input by planning, organizing, directing and controlling for the purpose of producing outputs desired by its customers so that organization objectives are accomplished.
49. Management is the guidance and control of action required to execute a program.
50. Management is the organizational process that includes strategic planning, setting objectives, managing resources, deploying the human and financial assets needed to achieve objectives, and measuring results.
51. Management is the activity of getting things done with the aid of people and other resources.

52. Management is the effective utilization and coordination of resources such as capital, plant, materials, and labor to achieve defined objectives with maximum efficiency.
53. Management is the process of getting activities completed efficiently with and through other people.
54. Management is the process of setting and achieving goals through the execution of five basic management functions: planning, organizing, staffing, directing, and controlling; that utilize human, financial, and material resources.
55. Management is a set of interactive processes through which the utilization of resources results in the accomplishment of organization objectives.
56. Management is the process of planning, leading, organizing and controlling people within a group in order to achieve goals.
57. Management is the process of achieving the objectives of the business organization by bringing together human, physical, and financial resources in an optimum combination and making the best decision for the organization while taking into consideration its operating environment.
58. Management is the organization and coordination of the activities of an enterprise in accordance with certain policies and in achievement of clearly defined objectives.
59. Management is the process of designing and maintaining an environment in which individuals, working together in groups, efficiently accomplish the objectives.
60. Management is defined as the purposeful and effective utilization of various resources for accomplishing a pre-determined objective.

An Administrator's Appeal

- Permit me the perspicacity to acknowledge that I can be no more effective than my subordinates enable me to be, and to deal with them so that they can help me by helping themselves.
- Courage me the consideration to recognize the worth of each individual and to respect all those with whom I have contact, neither stifling their development nor exalting myself at their expenses.
- Grant me the humility to learn from others, even though they be younger, less experienced, or of a humbler situation than I.
- Grant me the self-awareness to know honestly what I am, what I can do, and what I cannot.
- Permit me the patience to live realistically with my circumstances, striving always for the better, but recognizing the peril of a too rapid or a too drastic change.
- Grant me the judgment to channel my energies into those avenues which best utilize my abilities and do not require talents which I do not possess.
- Grant me the wisdom to cheerfully admit error and learn from my experiences, that I may grow and develop and avoid a repetition of mistakes.
- Concede me the courage to make decisions whenever they are necessary and to avoid rashness when they are not.
- Grant me the sensitivity to judge the reactions of others that I may modify my actions to meet the needs of those affected.
- Grant me the tolerance to recognize mistakes as the cost of true learning, and stand behind my subordinates, accepting my responsibility for their actions.
- Dare me the insight to develop a personal philosophy, so that my life may have more meaning and satisfaction and that I may avoid capricious action under the pressure of expediency.
- Allow me the all these things, dear Lord, that I may live a more useful life through the service of my fellow-men and through them serve Thee.

Keywords

Accident: An unexpected, unplanned occurrence which may involve injury or an unpremeditated event resulting in recognizable damage.

Accounting: The art of recording, classifying and summarizing in a significant manner and in terms of money transactions and events which are at least in part of financial character and interpreting the results thereof.

Acid Test Ratio: Sum of cash, marketable securities and receivables divided by current liabilities. It is also called quick ratio.

Accountability: It means to be answerable for one's conduct in respect to obligations fulfilled or unfulfilled.

Accreditation: It is a procedure by which an authoritative body gives formal recognition of technical competence of testing and or calibration for a laboratory to carry out specific tests.

Activity Limitation: Activity is the nature and extent of functioning at the level of the person. Activity may be limited in nature, duration and quality.

Admission: It is the acceptance of a patient by the hospital for inpatient service, which may be for investigations and or treatment.

Age-specific Fertility Rate: Number of live births in a year to 1000 women in any specified age group.

Allocate: To spread a cost from one account to several accounts, products, activities, or to several periods.

Ambulance: A vehicle for emergency care which carries equipment and supplies for optimal emergency care at the scene and during the period of transportation, to afford maximum safety and comfort and avoid aggravation of this condition.

Ambulatory Care: Outpatient care.

Appropriation: In governmental accounting, expenditure authorized for a specific purpose, amount and time.

Assessment: It is the testing and appraisal of trainees' performance or achievement, resulting from a training experience.

Assets: These are economic resources of an organization capable of being measured in monetary terms. These are cash, money claims, marketable securities, stock of materials, land, buildings, equipment, furniture, investment, patent, goodwill, copyright, etc.

Attack Rate: It is an incidence rate used when the population is exposed to risk for a limited period such as during an attack.

Attitude: A learned pre-disposition to respond in a consistently favorable or unfavorable manner with respect to a given object.

Audit: Systemic inspection of accounting records involving analyses, tests and confirmations, accomplished in accordance with auditing standards.

Authority: The sum of legitimate rights and powers entrusted to an individual to carry out his or her assigned responsibilities or duties.

Average Cost: This is a measure of total costs of production associated with each unit of output.

Average Daily Census: It is the average of patient in the hospital at a given time per day.

Average Length of Stay: It is the average number of days of service related to each discharged patient during the given period.

Balance Sheet: Statement of financial position which shows the assets, liabilities and owner's equity in an organization.

Bed Complement: It is the number of hospital beds normally available for use by the inpatient.

Biomedical Equipment: Equipments which are required for diagnostic, therapeutic and monitoring purposes for care and research purposes.

Biomedical Waste: Any waste which is generated during the diagnosis, treatment or immunization of human beings or animals or in research activities.

Birth Rate: The number of live births per 1000 estimated mid-year population in a given year.

Block Appointment: Calling for a certain number of patients to be present at given time.

Break Even Analysis: Comparison between cost and revenue to determine that volume of production where there is no loss, no profit for the organization.

Budget: It is a statement of plans expressed in quantitative, usually in financial term, covering specific period, usually one year.

Budgetary Control: The management of governmental and non-governmental unit in accordance with an official budget in order to keep total expenditures within authorized limits.

Budget Calendar: It lays down the specific dates for preparation, discussion and approval of departmental budget with a view to complete the entire budget exercise within the desired time.

Budget Committee: It receives reviews, coordinates departmental budgets into a total master budget and lays down the procedure for preparing and monitoring the budget.

Budgeting: Process of making a budget.

Budget Manual: A document which incorporates the statement of the general objectives and budget procedures and sets out the responsibilities of the persons engaged in the routine of and the form and records required for the budget control.

Budget Officer: An officer, who coordinates the preparation of the budget, monitors its progress, analyzes the variation by responsibility and cost centers and organizes follow-up action.

Budget Period: The duration for which budget is prepared and employed.

Business Process Re-engineering: The fundamental reconsideration and radical redesign of organizational processes, in order to achieve drastic improvement of current performance in cost, service and speed.

Business Transaction: Any exchange of money or money's worth as goods and services between two parties.

Camp Approach: It is a type of outreach program in which professional in rehabilitation field provide service to people with disabilities in neighboring area from time to time.

Capital: The stock of goods which are man-made and used in production.

Capital Account: Part of the balance of payments where flows of savings, investment and currency are recorded.

Capital Budget: It is the budget that is directed towards utilization of funds for the acquisition of fixed or long lived assets or new projects from which a stream of benefits is expected to be received during future years.

Capital Costs: These are usually defined as costs for items with a life of more than one year, e.g. costs of construction, equipment purchasing, etc.

Cash Budget: It is a summary of inflows and outflows over a period of time.

Centralization: It means that majority of decision about the work to be performed are not being made at the place of work or by those who perform the work but by those who are at higher levels.

Collective Bargaining: It is a method by which wage problems and conditions of employees are resolved amicably, peacefully and voluntarily between labor and management.

Communication: It is the process of transmitting information resulting in common understanding of all parties.

Community-based Rehabilitation: It is a strategy within the community for the development of the rehabilitation services, equalization of the opportunities and social integration of people with disabilities.

Community Health: It refers to the health status of the members of the community, to the problems affecting their health and to the totality of health care provided for the community.

Conflicts: It means opposition or disagreement between parties that calls for an agreement or a contract.

Consent: According to Indian Contract Act, section (13), two or more persons are said to consent when they agree upon the same thing in the same sense. Simply stated, it means voluntary agreement, compliance or permission.

Consumer: Any person who buys any goods or avails of any service, for a consideration which has been paid or promised to be paid; either fully or in some form of deferred payment.

Consumer Dispute: A dispute where a person against whom a complaint has been made denies the allegation.

Contribution: The difference between selling price and variable cost per unit.

Contribution Ratio: Contribution/selling price.

Coordination: It is the integrating process in an orderly pattern of group effort in any organization towards the accomplishment of the common objectives.

Cost: It is the sacrifice made in order to obtain a good or service.

Cost Accounting: It is a branch of accounting information system that records, measures and reports information about costs.

Cost Analysis: The process of rearranging the data in the existing accounts to obtain the cost of services rendered by the hospital.

Cost Benefit Analysis: It is a technique of economic evaluation that estimates the total costs and benefits of an activity in monetary terms.

Cost Control: Any activity aimed at ensuring the same benefit at the lowest cost or increasing the benefits without any further in cost.

Cost Effective Analysis: Method of analysis that estimates the cost associated with a particular technology/treatment in achieving given healthcare objectives. To become cost-effective, services/products should be defect-free.

Cost Minimization: It identifies the least cost intervention in achieving desired objectives.

Cost Utility Analysis: It is a form of cost effectiveness analysis but it measures effects of the project in terms of utilities.

Cost Volume Profit Analysis: It is a managerial tool to show the relationship between various components of profit planning, viz. cost, selling price and volume of activity.

Counseling: It is the process of helping a person to solve his problem by himself through advising and guiding.

Cross Price Elasticity of Demand: How demands reacts to change in the price of other products.

Central Sterile Services Department (CSSD): A department within a hospital where medical or surgical supplies and equipment are cleaned, prepared, processed, stored and issued for patient's use.

Current Account: Pare of balance of payments where payments for the purchase and sale of goods and services are recorded.

Current Ratio: Sum of current assets divided by a sum of current liabilities.

Day Care: A novel concept in health care by which a patient is admitted to the hospital for a few hours during the day for pre-planned surgery or diagnostic/treatment procedure. Such patient excluded from inpatient census.

Death: It is permanent disappearance of all evidence of life at any time after live birth has taken place.

Decentralization: It is the systemic effort to delegate to the lowest levels of all authority except that which is reserved to be exercised at central points.

Decision Making: The process of making choice from among several alternatives.

Decision Package: A document that identifies a specific activity in such a manner that management can evaluate it and rate it against other activities competing for the same or similar limited resources and decide whether to approve or disapprove it.

Delegation: Sharing or handling over of authority and responsibility to a subordinate.

Demand: It is the desire for a good combined with the willingness and ability to get the desire fulfilled.

Demand Curve: The relationship between demand and price is often portrayed as a demand curve.

Demography: Scientific study of human population.

Density of Population: The number of persons living per square kilometer.

Depreciation: Decrease in value of capital good because of passage of time, wear and tear, etc. An allowance for depreciation may be included as an operating cost in accounts.

Differentiation: The process by which the tasks and activities of an organization are segmented into smaller groups. The basis of differentiation may be function, product, location or customer.

Direct Patient Care Cost: Cost directly incurred or attributable to the patient care, e.g. Salary.

Disability: An existing difficulty in performing one or more activities, which in accordance with the subject's age sex and are normative social role are generally accepted as essential basic components of daily living.

Disaster: Any occurrence that causes damage, ecological disruption, loss of human life and deterioration of health and health services on a scale sufficient to warrant an extraordinary response from outside the affected community.

Discharge: It is the release of an inpatient. Death of an admitted patient is also considered as discharge.

Disinfection: It is a process distribution or removal of pathogen which gives rise to infection.

Economic Good: Goods which are scarce because their use has an opportunity cost.

Economies of Scale: The relationship between input and output as the scale of production increases can be represented on a scale.

Efficiency: Relates to output per unit cost of the resources employed. Resources are being used efficiently if a given output is produced at minimum cost, or maximum output is produced at a given cost.

Elasticity: The degree of responsiveness of one variable changes into another, if responsiveness is high; it is term as elastic; if low, inelastic.

Elasticity of Demand: It is the responsiveness of demand to change in variables.

Emergency: A condition determined clinically or perceived by the patient or attendants as requiring urgent medical services, failing which it could result in loss of life or limb.

Endowment Funds: Funds in which a donor has stipulated as a condition of his gift, that the principal of the fund is to be maintained inviolate and in perpetuity and that only income from investments of the fund may be expended.

Environment: The business environment of a firm comprising economic, social, political, cultural, legal and geographic factors which critically affect the working of organization.

Epidemic: It is the occurrence in a community or region of a number of cases of a disease that is usually large or unexpected for the given place and time.

Epidemic Curve: It is graph of the time distribution of epidemic cases.

Epidemiological Triad: It depicts the three factors—agent, host and environment essential for development of any disease. Disease can be prevented by removal of any one factor from the triad.

Epidemiology: Study of distribution and determinants of health related states and events in populations, and application of this study to control health problems.

Equipment Audit: Periodic evaluation of the quality of performance of equipment in a hospital.

Equipment Management: It refers to effective and purposeful utilization of equipment and maximizes their uptime and ensures efficiency, validity, reliability and safety of their day-to-day functioning.

Equity: A claim, which can be enforced against the assets of the firm.

Equity Ratio: Stockholder's equity divided by total assets.

Ergonomics: It is inter-disciplinary approach to interface between the worker, work place and the equipment.

Evaluation: It is a system designed to value the effects, effectiveness and efficiency of training and of trainer.

Expenditure: Outlay of money to purchase goods or services.

Expenses: The cost of earning revenues is called expenditure. Expenses occur when assets are consumed or liabilities are increased to produce revenues.

Expense Account: An account to accumulate expenses that is closed at the end of the accounting period.

Externalities: When the level of consumption or production of some good or service by a consumer or firm has a direct effect on the level of welfare of another consumer or firm, as opposed to indirect effect through the price mechanism. Certain activities have spillover effects on other producers or consumers.

Family Size: The total number of children a woman has born at a point in time.

Fertility: Actual bearing of children.

Finance: Provision of money as and when required.

Fiscal: To do with public expenditure and with raising government revenue, for instance through taxation.

Fixed Budget: A budget designed to remain unchanged irrespective of the level of activity.

Fixed Cost: Costs do not vary with the level of output in the considered time period. Remember: IRDA.

Flexible Budget: A budget designed to change in accordance with the level of activity actually attained.

Free Care or Charity Care: It represents services provided for which payment was never expected and for which the patient in not pursued.

Functional Limitation: Impairment may cause functional limitation which are partial or total inabilities to perform those activities necessary for motor, sensory or mental function within the range and manner of which a human being is normally capable, e.g. walking, speaking.

Functional Structure: The organization structure wherein activities and tasks are observed into smaller group of the basis of their belonging or contributing to a particular function such as manufacturing, marketing, etc.

Fund Statement: An informal name often used for the statement of changes in financial position.

Gross Domestic Product (GDP): Measure of national income before property income from abroad and depreciation have been accounted for.

Gross National Product (GNP): A measure of national income including net property income from abroad but before depreciation.

General Fertility Rate: Number of live births per 1000 women in the reproductive age-group (15–44 or 49 years) in a given year.

General Marital Fertility Rate: Number of live births per 1000 married women in the reproductive age group (15–44 or 49 years) in a given year.

Geographical Structure: The organization structure in which activities and tasks are grouped together on the basis of their location in a geographical zone.

Grievance: A generic term covering the processes and methods through which members of the workforce may express disagreement with the conditions of employment.

Gross Death: Total deaths of hospitalized patients.

Gross Profit: This is the difference between the sales and cost of goods and services provided.

Gross Reproduction Rate: Average number of girls that would be born to a woman of she experiences the current fertility pattern throughout her reproductive span (15–44 or 49 years), assuming no mortality.

Group: Two or more persons who are interacting with one another in such a manner that each person influences and is influenced by each other person.

Group Cohesiveness: Attachment of members with the group.

Group Norms: Group behavior, standard beliefs, attitudes, traditions, expectation shared by group members.

HAI (Nosocomial infection): Infection acquired by the person in the hospital, manifestation of which may occur during hospitalization or after discharge from the hospital.

Handicap: A disadvantage for a given individual, resulting from an impairment or a disability, that limits or prevents the fulfillment of a role that is normal for that individual.

Hazards: A situation of risk or danger to health and safety.

Health: A state of complete physical, mental and social well-being and not merely an absence of disease or infirmity (WHO definition of health).

Health Care: Multitude of services rendered to individuals, families or communities by the agents of the health services or professions, for the purpose of promotion, maintaining, monitoring or restoring health.

Health Development: The process of continuous progressive improvement of the health status of a population.

Health Economics: An application of the theories, techniques and concepts of economics to the health sectors.

Health Financing: It means raising of resources to pay for goods or services.

Health for All: It means health is to be brought within the reach of everyone in a given community.

Health Information System: A mechanism for the collection, progressing, analysis and transmission of information required for organizing and operating health services and also for research and training.

Health Marketing: It involves in creating, communicating, and delivering health information and interventions using customer-centered and science-based strategies to protect and promote the health of diverse populations.

Health Promotion: The process of enabling people to increase control over, and to improve health.

Health Protection: The provision of conditions for normal mental and physical functioning of the human being individually and in group. It includes the promotion of health, the prevention of disease and curative and restorative medicine in all its aspects.

Hierarchy: A body classified in successively subordinate grades.

Hospital: It is an integral part of a social and medical organization, the function of which is to provide for the population complete health care, both curative and preventive, and whose outpatient services reaches out to the family and its home environment. The hospital is also a center for the training of health workers and bio-social research. (WHO definition of Hospital).

Hospital Census: Total numbers of inpatients occupying beds in the hospital at the census taking hours.

Hospital Death: Death of an admitted patient.

Hospital Housekeeping Management: It is a branch of general management which deals with cleanliness of the hospital, general environmental hygiene, sanitation and disposal of waste using appropriate methods, materials and manpower.

Hospital Linen: All clothings made of cotton, linen or wool or synthetic fabrics which are used by the patient or for the patient.

Hospital Waste: All waste generated, discarded and not intended for further use in the hospital.

Hotel Cost: These are costs, such as catering, laundry and linen that are incurred for each patient day in the hospital.

Human capital: Human skills and capabilities generated by investments in education and health (WHO).

Human Resources Development: It refers to functions involved in planning, managing and supporting the professional development of the health workforce within a health system, both at the strategic and policy levels.

Human Resources Planning: Process of estimating potential requirements for human resources in health and of designing ways of fulfilling those requirements.

Human Resource Policies: Guidelines and directions that regulate the utilization of workforce both within the health sector and within the wider context.

Impairment: It is a loss or abnormality of body structure or of a physiological or psychological function.

Immunity: The body is able to recognize, destroy and eliminate foreign antigens by producing specific or nonspecific antibodies against the foreign antigen. This ability of the body to protect self and destroy the invaders is called as—Immunity.

Incidence: The number of new cases occurring in a define population during a specified period of time.

Income Elasticity of Demand: How demand reacts to change in income.

Incremental Budget: It is the traditional and commonly used approach of budgeting wherein the previous year expending level is extrapolated for the next year and the incremental for processes, material and inflation is added.

Incubation Period: Time that elapses between the entry of the living agent to the appearance of the first sign and symptoms of the concerned disease.

Indifferent Analysis: It is an alternative way of explaining consumer choice that does not require an explicit discussion on utility.

Indirect Patient Care Cost: Cost indirectly incurred or not directly attributable to the patient care.

Individual Appointment: Calling for a certain patient to be present at a given time.

Induction: It means introducing an employee to the job and to the organization.

Industrial Dispute: Any dispute between employees and employees or employers and employers or employees and employers which is connected with the employment or non-employment or the terms of employment or with the condition of labor of any person.

Infection: The entry of disease producing agents in animal or human being where they multiply and develop and produce a subclinical, clinical disease state or a carrier state.

Input: Various resources such as men, money and material available for production capacity.

Integration: The process by which differentiated groups are pulled together to contribute towards the common organizational objectives. Hierarchical control, administrative procedure and communication networks are the process used for integration.

Intelligent Building: This is defined to anticipate the needs of the owner and occupant and possesses the ability to apply knowledge, act fast, think fast and learn.

Intensive Care Unit: A specific area of the hospital where sophisticated monitoring, titrated life support, specific therapy and specialized nursing, can be best provided for potentially salvageable, critically ill patient with life-threatening illness or injury.

Internal Audit: An audit conducted by employees to ascertain that internal control procedures are working or not.

Internal Control: The procedures used by a business in attempting to ensure that operations are carried out or recorded as planned.

Internal Marketing: Application of marketing, human resource management and allied theories, techniques and principles to manage, mobilize and motivate the employees at all levels of the organization to continuously improve the way they service external customers and each other.

Intervention: Any attempt to intervene or interrupt the usual sequence in the development of disease in human being.

Inventory: Idle resources of any kind having an economic value.

Inventory Control: It is a scientific process by which an organization is supplied with the goods and services, that it needs to achieve its objective at optimum cost.

Inventory Turnover: Number of times the average inventory has been sold during a period. Used to determine the effectiveness of inventory management.

Job Analysis: Process of identifying the requirements and defining roles of specific tasks.

Job Description: The scope of job activities, major responsibilities and positioning of the job in the organization.

Job Satisfaction: The amount of overall positive feelings that individuals have towards their jobs.

Job Specification: A list of various qualities which the individual doing the job should possess.

Laboratory: It is a place of work for testing patient sample for results in favor of diagnostic and treatment.

Labor Legislation: Policies and guidelines regulating the labor market. Laws and regulations that govern the functioning of the labor market.

Labor Relations: Relations between management and employees in relation to collective bargaining and maintenance of contract.

Laparoscopic Surgery: Major surgical interventions are done with the help of laparoscope. Its use requires minimal incision, postoperative care and stay in the hospital.

Law of Agency: This states that the acts of the purchaser done within the apparent scope of his authority binds his hospital with respect to third parties, in respect of any contract concluded.

Law of Contract: A formal contract of purchase duly signed by an authorized hospital purchaser binds both the seller and the buyer. An offer becomes a contract only when it is accepted by the seller.

Law of Demand: According to law of demand, other things being equal, if the price of a commodity falls, the quantity demanded of it will rise and if the price of a commodity rises, its quantity demanded will decline. There is inverse relationship between price and quantity demanded.

Law of Supply: Other things remain constant; the quantity of good produced and offered for sale will increase as the price of the good rises and decrease as the price falls.

Lay-off, Downsizing, Redundancies: Staff reductions resulting from organizational changes or budget cuts; form of termination of employment without negative evaluation of performance.

Leadership: It is a process of encouraging and influencing the people to direct their efforts towards the achievement of some particular goals in a given situation.

Lead Time: It is the length of time in days between the decision to replenish an item and its actual addition to stock.

Learning: Relatively permanent change in behavior that occurs as a result of experience or reinforced practice.

Ledger: Individual accounts of persons, property and assets, expenses, incomes, etc. are opened in another book called ledger.

Life Expectancy: The average number of years which a person of that age may expect to live according to the mortality pattern prevalent in that country.

Line Function: Any function which directly contributing to the organization's objectives.

Liabilities: These are economic obligations of an organization to pay cash or to provide goods or services in some future period. These are creditors, bills payable, wages and salaries payable, interest, taxes, bonds, debenture, loans, etc.

Liquidity: A firm's cash position and its ability to meet obligations as they mature.

Lock-out: It means a temporary closing of a place of establishment or the suspension of work or the refusal by the employer to continue to employ any number of persons employed by him.

Logistic Management: The process of planning, implementing and controlling the efficient, effective flow and storage of goods, services and related information from point of origin to point of consumption for the purpose of conforming to customer requirement.

Maintenance: It is an essential function of service management that is concerned with day-to-day problems keeping the hospital in good functioning condition.

Manpower Planning: A strategy for the acquisition, utilization, improvement and preservation of the human resource of an organization.

Marginal Cost: The change in total cost at a given scale of output when a little more or little less output is produced.

Marketing: The process of planning and executing the conception, pricing, promotion and distribution of ideas, goods and services to create exchanges that satisfy individual and or organizational goals.

Marketing Mix: It is a term used to describe the integration of four fundamental marketing elements, which are sometimes called the 'four Ps': Product, Price, Place and Promotion.

Market Segmentation: The process of dividing a market into meaningful, relatively similar and identifiable segment or groups.

Master or Final Budget: This is a summary budget which incorporates all financial budgets in a capsule form.

Material Management: Process of management which coordinates, supervises and executes the tasks associated with the flow of material to, through and out of an organization in an integrated manner.

Matrix Structure: Used generally for project execution which requires the services of skilled functional people and the specialized knowledge of product specialists. It is a combination of the functional and product structures and its distinguishing characteristic is dual authority.

Medical Emergency: A situation when the patient required urgent and high quality medical care to prevent loss of life and limbs and initiate the action for restoration of normal healthy life.

Medical Audit: Evaluation of medical care in retrospective through analysis of clinical records.

Medical Record: A clinical, scientific, administrative and legal document relating to patient care in which are recorded sufficient data written in sequence of events to justify the diagnosis, warrant the treatment and results.

Medicolegal Case: A medicolegal case is defined as one, where an attending doctor, after taking the history and examination of the patient, thinks that some investigation by the law enforcing agencies are required so as to fix responsibility regarding the case in accordance with the law of the land.

Microsurgery: Surgery performed under magnification.

Monitoring: It is a function of management which measures the changes during the implementation of a program and it checks the progress to see if activities take place as scheduled.

Monopolistic Competition: Market structure where a large number of small firms produce non-homogeneous products and where there are no barriers to entry or exit.

Monopoly: The control of the supply of a product or service by one person or organization only.

Motivation: It is a process that starts with physiological or psychological deficiency or need that activates behavior or drive that is aimed at goals or incentive.

Negotiation: It is essentially a discussion between a buyer and a seller with a view to reaching an agreement.

Net Death: Total death after 48 hours of admission.

Net Income: The amount by which the total revenue earned during the accounting period exceeds total expenses incurred during the same period.

Net Profit: Profit after paying the tax.

Network Structure: A structure in which one organization acts as the lead organization and creates a network of many other external organizations whose services the lead organization utilizes in fulfillment of its objectives.

Non-operating Expenses: Expenses incurred in generating the non-operating revenues.

Non-operating Revenues: Revenues which are incidental to the main operations of the business, e.g. sale of old instruments.

Nursing Audit: Periodic evaluation of nursing service (PENS).

Nursing Care: The conscious practice of human relationships.

Nursing Record: The record of events pertaining to patients, maintain by a nursing personnel.

Nursing Service: A WHO expert committee on nursing defines the Nursing Service as that part of total health organization which aims to satisfy the nursing needs of the community.

Obsolete Materials: Those items which are not required at all due to changes in design or models.

Occupancy Rate: It is the ratio of actual patient days expressed as a percentage of the maximum possible patient days during any given period.

Occupational Disease: Disease known to arise out of exposure to substances and dangerous conditions in processes, trades or occupations.

Oligopoly: Limited competition between two large companies.

Operating Cost or Recurrent Cost: Cost of operating an enterprise or service.

Operating Expenses: These are the expenses relating to main operations of the business firm, e.g. depreciation.

Operating Profit: Profit before interest and tax, which is a measure of performance of firm operations.

Operating Revenues: Revenues generating from the actual operation of a business firm, e.g. OPD collection.

Operational Efficiency: Producing given output at minimum cost or maximizes output for given cost.

Operation or Non-planned Budget: It is the budget that is directed towards utilization of funds for achieving short-term operational goals.

Operations Management: Activities necessary to produce and deliver a product/service.

Operation Research: The application of scientific methods to the study of alternatives in a problem situation, in order to obtaining a quantitative basis for arriving at a best possible solution.

Opportunity Cost: Economic cost of production, benefit lost from the next best alternative.

Organization: It refers to all types of formal bodies created for a specific purpose.

Organizational Behavior: It is an interdisciplinary field dedicated to better understanding and managing people at work (study of human behavior).

Organizational Culture: The set of values that defines for members what the organization stands for, how it operates and what it considers important.

Organizational Climate: A set of characteristics and factors that are perceived by the employees about their organizations which serve as a major force in influencing their behavior.

Organizational Design: It is the overall configuration of structural components that defines jobs, groups of jobs, the hierarchy, patterns of authority, and approaches to coordination and line-staff differentiation into a single, unified organizational system.

Organizational Development: A technique for bringing change in the entire aspect of the organization, rather than focusing attention on individuals, so that change is easily absorbed.

Organizational Effectiveness: The degree to which organization realizes its goals. It is the extent to which an organization, given certain resources and means, achieves its objectives without placing undue strain on its members.

Organizational Objective: The specific purposes, results and achievements sought by the organization.

Organization Chart: The depiction of specific positions in an organization, their states within the organization and the reporting relationship between a subordinate and his superior.

Outpatient: A person given diagnostic, therapeutic or preventive services through the hospital facilities and is not registered as an inpatient at a time.

Outbreak: A smaller epidemic in the interest of minimizing public alarm.

Outsourcing: It means that products and services are contracted to outside vendors that have expertise in a particular area.

Overhead Cost: All indirect costs are overhead costs.

Owner's Equity: The financial interest of the owner in monetary term is called owner's equity. It is the difference of the assets minus liabilities.

Participation Restriction: Participation is the nature and extent of a person's involvement in life situation in relationship to impairments, activities, health conditions and contextual factors.

Patient Day: Number of patients for whom lodging and other services have been provided in the hospital between two successive census taking hours.

Perception: It is an important mediating cognitive process of organizing, selection and interpreting environmental information.

Perfect Competition: Market structure where there are many buyers and sellers, where there is freedom of entry and exit to the market, perfect knowledge, and where all firms produce a homogeneous product.

Performance Budget: The process of analyzing, identifying, simplifying and crystallizing specific performance objectives of a job to be achieved over a period in the framework of the organizational objectives.

Personality: A stable set of characteristics and tendencies that determine those communalities and differences in the psychological behavior and that may not be easily understood as the sole result of the social and biological pressures of the moment.

Pharmacy: The department which deals with all aspect of drugs except prescribing and administration, which are exclusively right of the physicians and nurses respectively.

Planning: It is deciding in advance what to do, how to do it, when to do it, who is to do it. It bridges the gap from where we are to where we want to go.

Playback Period: Amount of time that must elapse before the cash inflows from a project equal the cash outflows.

Power: It is the potential ability of a person or group to influence another person or group.

Presumptive Treatment: Antimalarial treatment given on assumption that all fever cases are due to malaria, administered before blood film is examined.

Prevalence: It refers specifically to all current cases existing in a given population at a given point of time.

Preventive Maintenance: This pertains to critical system maintenance to reduce the possible risk of failures to a minimum, parts and sub-systems which are suspected to be unreliable are replaced before they actually fail, thus ensuring high reliability but at extra cost.

Price Elasticity of Demand: How demand reacts to change in price.

Price Elasticity of Supply: How sensitive quantity supplied is to change in the price of the product.

Primary Health Care: It is essential health care based on practical, scientifically sound and socially acceptable methods and technology made universally accessible to individuals and families in the community through their full participation and at a cost that the community and country can afford to maintain at every stage of their development in the spirit of self-determination.

Primary Prevention: Action taken prior to the onset of the disease, which removes the possibility that a disease will occur, e.g. immunization.

Primordial Prevention: Prevention of the emergence or development of risk factors in countries or population groups in which they have not yet appeared.

Principle of Division of Work: That principle by which work is organized into smaller jobs allowing people to undertake only specialized activities thus ensuring efficiency in the use of labor.

Principle of Span of Control: The principle which states that there is a limit in each managerial position on the number of persons which can be effectively controlled.

Privileged Communication: A communication made by a doctor to the proper authority who is corresponding legal, social and moral duties to protect the public.

Process: Describes the transformation/productive technique which changes input into desired outputs.

Product Structure: An organization in which activities and the tasks are grouped on the basis of individual products.

Production: It is the process of producing goods or services which satisfy human wants.

Productive Efficiency: Production is at lowest cost.

Professional Secret: This is the one which a doctor comes to know in his professional capacity while dealing with the patient.

Profit: Difference between the sales revenues and total costs.

Profit before Tax: This is the figure after deducting interest from PBT.

Public Health: It is a science which involves methods to prevent diseases and improve the well-being of the general public.

Quality: Inherent characteristic and distinctive attribute that makes a product/service different from others.

Quality Circles: These are the small groups of workers who meet regularly with their supervisor as the circle leader to solve work-related problems.

Quality Control: The operational techniques and activities that are used to fulfill requirements of quality. It is a statistical system for measuring reproducibility of degree of precision in laboratory procedure.

Quality Manual: A document stating the mission and vision of the organizations as to the quality, the quality policy and describing the quality system of an organization.

Quality of Care: The degree to which health services for individuals and populations increase the likelihood of desire health outcomes and are consistent with current professional knowledge.

Quality of Service: Totality of features and characteristics of service that bears on its ability to satisfy stated and implied need of its patient.

Quality of Work Life: An attempt through a formal program to integrate employee needs and well-being with the intention of improved productivity, greater worker involvement and higher level of job satisfaction.

Radical Treatment: Antimalarial treatment given to the blood film positive cases during follow-up visit.

Real Account: Balance sheet account as opposed to nominal or income account.

Recruitment: It is a process of identifying the prospective persons, stimulating and encouraging them to apply for a particular post in the organization.

Remuneration: Payment of an equivalent to a person for a service or expense.

Reorder Level: This denotes the stock level at which a fresh order has to be placed. This is equal to average consumption per day multiplied by lead time plus the safety stock.

Reservoir of Infection: Any part of living or inanimate environment which harbors the pathogenic organism capable of being transmitted to humans and animals.

Reserve/Buffer/Safety Stock: It is the minimum quantity of supply set apart as an insurance against variation in supply and demand.

Responsibility: It refers to duties that is those mental and physical activities which an individual is required to perform by virtue of his membership in the organization.

Revenues: These are the benefits that the customers contribute to an organization in exchange for goods and services provided by it.

Revolving Fund: A fund whose amounts are continually expended and then replenished; for example, a petty cash fund.

Rehabilitation: Combined and coordinated use of medical, social, educational and vocational measures for training and retraining the individual to the highest level of functional ability.

Scalar Principle: The chain of direct authority relationship from superior to subordinate within the organization.

Secondary Prevention: Action which halts the progress of the disease at its incipient stage and prevents complications.

Selection: Rejecting applicant by choosing and examining.

Self-balancing: A set of records with equal debits and credits such as the balance sheet, and a fund in non-profit accounting.

Services: An activity or series of activities of more or less intangible nature that normally, not necessarily take place in interaction between the customer and service.

Service Marketing: Activity or benefit that one party can offer to another that is essentially intangible and does not result in the ownership of anything. Its production may or may not be tied to a physical product.

Service Quality: It is the delivery of excellent or superior service relative to the customer expectations.

Sex Ratio: The number of females per 1000 males.

Staff Function: Functions which are advisory or auxiliary in nature but do not directly contribute towards the organizational objectives.

Sterilization: A process of freeing an article from all living organisms including bacteria, virus and fungal spores.

Strategy: The chosen path from among several alternative paths evolved and evaluated to achieve an already established objective.

Strategic Alliance: It refers to aligning with a potential or real fellow competitor to forge a front in order to effectively deal with the environmental opportunities and threats by augmenting the front's collective strength and eliminating weakness.

Stress: It is the reactions of individuals to new or threatening factors in their work environment.

Structure: Formal and established pattern of relationship in an organization.

Supervision: The effort to stimulate, coordinate and guide the continued growth of the hospital staff both individually and collectively.

Supply: This is what the seller is able and willing to offer for sale.

Supply Chain Management: This is the management of two way flow of manpower, money, material, equipment and information within and among organization to ensure the efficient and fast delivery of goods and services to the end customer.

Surplus Materials: Those materials which have no immediate use but have accumulated due to faulty planning, forecasting and purchasing.

Synergy: Cooperation of two or more things to produce combined effects greater than the sum of their separate effects.

System: A particular linking of inter-related and inter-dependent components having a facilitating effect on the carrying out of one or more processes.

Techniques of Economic Evaluation: The quantitative analysis of the relative desirability to the whole community of investigating in alternative projects.

Tertiary Prevention: All measures available to reduce or limit impairments and disabilities and minimize suffering caused by existing disability.

Total Cost: It is a measure of all the costs entailed in producing a given level of output. It is derived by summing up all the costs incurred during production.

Total Quality Management: A management approach of an organization centered on quality, based on participation of all its members and aiming at long-term success through customer satisfaction and benefits to all members of the organization and to society. It is one of the most promising managerial innovations which increase the efficiency and effectiveness of healthcare services.

Trade Union: Any combination of person whether temporary or permanent formed for the purpose of employees and employees or employers and employers or employees and employers; or imposing restrictive condition on the conduct of any trade or business and includes federation of two or more trade unions.

Training: It is the process of developing skills, knowledge and changing attitudes, so as to increase individual and organizational effectiveness.

Transformational Leadership: This is a leadership that transmits a sense of mission, stimulates learning experiences and inspires ways of thinking. Also known as charismatic leadership, inspirational leadership, symbolic leadership.

Treatment: It is the process by which waste is modified before it is finally disposed off, so that it can no more act as a source of pathogen.

Treatment Cost: These are case dependent costs associated with a particular diagnostic, therapeutic and other treatment/services provided to the patient.

Trial Balance: A listing of account balance. All accounts with debit balances are totally separated from accounts with credit balances. The two totals should be equal.

Turnover: It means total trading income from cash sales and credit sales.

Unity of Command: It means that employees should receive orders from one superior only.

Utility: Satisfaction derived from consuming a good.

Utilization Index: It is the parameter to assess the productivity of service or equipment.

Value Analysis: An organized innovative approach which has its objective—the achievement of the value of the product. Value analysis aims at reducing the cost value to the value of the products.

Variable Cost: These are the costs which vary according to the volume of production.

Voucher: A document that recognizes a liability and authorizes the disbursement of the cash.

Vulnerability: Something that could lead to injury, harm or threat to person, property, ideals or image.

Wages: All remuneration, including salary, allowances or otherwise expressed in term of money or capable of being so expressed, which would, if the terms employment express or implied were fulfilled be payable to a person employed in respect to his employment.

Wage Period: According to Payment of Wage Act, 1936 section (4), employer is bound to fixed wage period. Wage period may fix as payable—daily, weekly, fortnightly or monthly. No wage period shall exceed one month.

Working Capital: Current assets. It can also mean net working capita which is current assets minus current liabilities.

Word of Mouth or Mouth Publicity: Oral, person to person communication between a receiver and a communicator whom the receiver perceives as non-commercial regarding a brand, a product or a service.

Working Conditions: Characteristics of the environment in which a person is expected to work. Includes terms of employment, benefits, physical and social climate.

Zero-based Budgeting: It is an operational planning and budgeting process which requires each manager to justify the entire budget request in detail from scratch and shift the burden of proof to each manager to justify why he should spend any money at all.

Management Mantra

- Management is made up of four M: Men, Money, Material and Machine.
- Managerial issue means application of management tools to ensure effective and efficient functioning of the organization.
- No issue is settled until it is settled right.
- Manage men, men will manage everything.
- Every problem has its own solution and control.
- Service should be dynamic, qualitative and cost-effective.
- Maintain cordial relationship with others.
- A leader is one who knows the way, shows the way and goes the way.
- A quality report and customer satisfaction is the final goal of evaluation.
- HR is one of the most important and live input of any organization.
- No machine is ever useful without its operator.
- What for Whom—is the basic question for planning an activity.
- No organization can grow till its all members are satisfied to the desire level of satisfaction.
- The ultimate aim of any service is to achieve its desired objective with full satisfaction of customer and provider.
- In today's high-tech world, even super computer remains a showpiece till well-developed software is developed and fed in.
- Morale of the staff irrespective of his status directly effects organization, environment and culture and in turns its output.
- The staff selection, positioning, satisfaction and their training is very important aspect to achieve desire results of the department.
- An orientation program is one of the most overlooked management tool.
- Opportunities always flavor prepared mind!
- Everything can be done better than it is being done.
- Efficiency is not everything.
- A decision which does not result in action is meaningless.
- Self-discipline is the best discipline and it is attitude of mind.
- Public always demanding more and better service at minimum cost.
- The greatest failure is not to try!
- Training is required to learn new techniques and concept.
- Policies are general guidelines for decision making.
- Effective management is always situational management.
- Kite rises against the wind.

- A man should be like his tea; his real strength appearing when he gets into hot water.
- Singleness of purpose is one of the chief essential for success in life.
- The only thing more expensive than education is ignorance.
- Leadership is doing the right thing in the right manner at the right time as a matter of right.
- Human life cannot measured in monetary term.
- Customer focus is the prime requirement for quality management program.
- The major concern of administration is with the art of getting thing done.
- Collective bargaining is an important means of maintaining industrial peace.
- Even small thing makes perfection and perfection is not small thing.
- Cost analysis is cost accounting technique.
- Objective of training is to achieve a clearly defined performance.
- To create a surplus is the ultimate goal of all managers.
- Management is an art of getting thing done through people.
- Cost volume profit analysis includes the entire process of profit planning whereas break-even analysis is widely used techniques to study this process.
- SERVE, it means, Safety, Efficiency, Reliability, Validity, and Effectiveness.
- Problem is identified by the difference between what is actually happening in a situation and what one wishes to have occurred.
- Teams are built, not born.
- Administration makes its greatest contribution in second managerial function, i.e. organizing.
- Management is defined in a simple term is to get the work done in a systemic way for accomplishment of defined objectives based on management of man, money and material.
- Management is a process by which a cooperative group directs action towards common goals.
- Management of men is not an easy job.
- Coordination is one of the most important managerial functions.
- Things easy to get yesterday may be difficult to get tomorrow and vice-versa.
- Quality makes the difference.
- Service should be essentially defecting free.
- He that plants thorns must never expect to gather roses.

- To become cost-effective product should be defect-free.
- Promotional avenue having some motivational value.
- Negotiation is nothing but a discussion between buyer and seller with a view to reaching an agreement.
- Quality is the inherent characteristic and distinctive attribute that makes a product different from others.
- Security staff should not be part of the union.
- Items which have no immediate use but stored due to faulty planning, forecasting and purchasing is labeled as surplus.
- Scrap, surplus and obsolete items are problematic for the management.
- Inventory control deals with physical control of inventories.
- One Man Makes the Difference....The leader.
- Cost accounting is the account of cost.
- Finance is the life of an organization.
- Management is the process by which an organization employs its resources to achieve pre-determined objectives.
- Profit is nothing but the difference between revenue and expenses.
- Accounting is the language of business.
- Reliability does not guarantee certainty in decision making.
- Debit the receiver and credit the giver.
- Expenses, income and losses are formal fictitious account.
- Cost is the sacrifice made in order to obtain a good or service.
- Knowledge is empowering!
- To provide quality services, an organization first should first learn about consumer expectation through market research.
- Communication is an essential part of marketing.
- Remember you are not alone in the market to provide services.
- Quality of service is very difficult to judge.
- Finance is provision of money as and when required.
- Marketing research is the objective and systemic process of gathering, analyzing and interpreting data relevant to a specific situation or problem facing an institution.
- *Secret of good administrator:* Dedication, devotion, and hard work.
- Price refers to money value that the customer has to pay.
- Pricing of service require separate treatment than pricing of goods.
- Mass production is not possible in service.
- 100% pure product is not possible.
- Services are generally produced and consumed at the same time.
- Quality is become an essential part of service marketing.
- Marketing covers wide range of critical business activities.

- Inventories proportional to problems and cost.
- Basic principle of inventory control is to contain cost.
- Cost of not having the items sometimes costlier than cost of having.
- Larger is the inventories greater are the problems.
- Discard any items when it became BERU—Beyond economic repair, unserviceable.
- Equipment functioning effectively, safely and life-long, if maintain properly.
- Keep your business in your own hand. It is the only way to be happy.
- Material which not moving for 2 or 3 years is declared as surpluses.
- Take the problem as an opportunity.
- Inventory control is one of the modern management techniques of operation research.
- Inventories are yard of business.
- An idle resource of any kind having an economic value is called inventory.
- Without proper inventory control, problems related to manufacturing, marketing, money and motto can be precipitate.
- Motivate all the staff to contain cost.
- Training is essential to develop to do a good job in a minimum time with minimum cost and maximum effects.
- People forget, records remember.
- Outsourcing enhances quality of service.
- Contracting reduces cost, responsibility and workload of the management.
- Little drop of water make the mighty ocean.
- No safety program is complete without training and awareness.
- As the world becomes noisier, it becomes less meaningful.
- No energy is more expensive than no energy.
- Gardening is the great asset in reducing dust and noise.
- An intelligent building is one that is designed to anticipate the need of the owner and the occupant, and possesses the ability to learn, think fast, apply knowledge and act fast.
- Need-based training will definitely improve the technical performance of the employee.
- Right people are the future of the organization.
- A determination to succeed is the only way to succeed.
- Always plan for future.
- Meaning of words is not in words, they are within us.

- Studies have shown that concentration of the learner starts dipping after 20–25 minutes, even if lecture is interesting.
- No organization can survive without manpower.
- Manpower is the main power in any organization.
- Manpower gap is the difference between demand and supply of manpower.
- Successful communication is the transfer of meaning and understanding between two people.
- Good communication is the foundation for sound management.
- Any breakdown in communication could be costly.
- It is impossible to have human relations without communication.
- Average executive spends nearly 70% of his time in communication.
- A message could be oral, written, telephonic, face-to-face, mass-media.
- Evaluation of training is needed for valuation of training.
- Training should be result oriented.
- Research shows that the ability of learning remain unimpaired throughout life.
- Motivational level can also be increased by training.
- Matching the right people with the right job is the biggest challenge for manpower.
- Motivation is the master key of management.
- Managing people is the key to success in any system.
- Authority can be fully delegated while responsibility can only be partially delegated.
- Careful read the situation and then be flexible enough to adapt.
- Put yourself in the shoes of the subordinate.
- Management is the practice of consciously and continually shaping of an organization.
- Management meant more than just—what was happening inside a particular organization.
- Without effective management, organization is likely to get into difficulties.
- Without a goal, no organization would have a reason to exist.
- Anyone who plans to make a living in a organization needs to study organizational behavior.
- Human engineering deals with study of people at work and of work method.
- A satisfied employee is a hard working one.
- The Japanese are world leader because of their emphasis on quality.

- Management principles and theories are mainly the product of rigorous scientific methodology.
- Management can be both a science and art.
- Management must be decision maker.
- Decision making is a process of choosing between alternative courses of action.
- To make a decision you require information.
- Budget is a traditional and widely used control process.
- Money is the most commonly used motivating factor.
- Job satisfaction is the most important motivating factor.
- One man makes the difference that is a leader.
- Performance appraisal to evaluate how the person performs in his particular job.
- Service cannot be stored, resold or returned.
- Appraiser should be capable of determining what is more important and what is relatively less important.
- Operation research is the application of scientific method to manage problems.
- A network diagram of activity is the key feature of PERT and acts as a ROAD MAP to reach the objectives.
- Goal must be SMART, it means, Specific, Measurable, Achievable, Relevant, and Time bound.
- MBO is nothing but appraisal by result.
- Manager must possess technical skills, human skills, and conceptual skills.
- Be aware of the defects and repair them with every glowing and conscientious observation, be blessed and make others blessed too.
- Trauma is one of the biggest killers in the world.
- To attend roadside accident victims is the legal and moral duty of every citizen.
- We have to preserve the earth for the future generation.
- Human element is more important than any technology.
- All things do not mean the same to all men.
- Leader is a person who can motivate a group of people to achieve the task and maintain team unity throughout the process.
- Right to life means life with dignity.
- Work with people rather than to use them.
- As a manager, participative approach is often more appropriate particularly when working with other professionals.

- Through proper motivation, productivity increased and conflict can be avoided.
- Leadership transforms potential into reality.
- There is no best way to influence people.
- Manager spends about 60–90% of the working day on communication.
- Human resources are more valuable than any other resources, and that their proper management can tremendously help the organizations to maximize the utilization of other resources.
- Human relations are supreme importance in any organization.
- Employees, knowledge, skills, and attitude need to be respected.
- Training in communication and motivation helps a lot in building human relations.
- The dictionary meaning of "Policy" is a plan of action and that "Plan" is a policy.
- If you do not have a plan for pleasure, you will have pain.
- Authority is ineffective without ability to exercise it.
- Motivation is goal directed behavior.
- Motivation is a Latin word, meaning to move.
- Staff is a real strength of any organization, so take care of them.
- Time is of essence.
- Inventory is an idle resource of any kind.
- Machine selected should be user friendly.
- HRD is essential for any organization that would like to be dynamic and growth oriented.
- People perform better when they feel trusted and see meaning in what they are doing.
- Training is linked with performance appraisal and career development.
- Rewarding employee performance and behavior is an important part of HRD.
- Without evaluation, administration becomes an unfinished business.
- Motivation includes self-motivation and motivation of others.
- Manager must spend considerable time in negotiations, with outside agency and the staff within.
- Important areas for evaluation are employees.
- Multiple responsibilities produce several kinds of conflicts.
- Sustainable development cannot be achieved without paying proper attention to HRD function.
- About 90% of the decisions made in an organization are of routine variety.

- Good judgment is needed to increase the possibility of desired outcomes and minimize the possibility of undesired outcomes.
- Security and motivation tremendously add to success rate.
- The most important thing in HRD is creating a climate of trust and development.
- Health is a fundamental human right and a basic need.
- Fine goals matter less than the right strategy.
- Training is one of the important aspects of manpower development.
- Training should be need based.
- You cannot be expert in everything. You do not have to. But you should know who are the experts in each area and be able to call upon their advice when needed.
- Ideas not acted upon are useless.
- India is the largest democracy in the world.
- More you sweat in peace, less you bleed in war.
- NEWS stand for Nutrition, Education, Water, and Shelter—are essential requirement for well-being.
- Management techniques are applied scientifically and methodically for success of any enterprise.
- Pre-planning prevents poor performance.
- It is better to be dressed homely neat, than to be abnormally gorgeous.
- Service quality is essentially what customer perceives.
- To understand the situation is first important aspect to manage the situation.
- India is one of the most disaster-prone countries.
- *Disaster:* Be prepared.
- Management is the process whereby those unrelated resources are integrated into a total system of objective accomplishment.
- People is considered as the most important and vital variable in the organization.
- Automation is the greatest industry.
- No one can prevent the technology.
- Public interest should always be protected.
- Image of any organization does not develop on its own but much strategic planning is required with amalgamation of science and art.
- Focus on bad system rather than bad staff.
- Research is essentially an attitude of mind and the application of a technique in confronting a problem.
- An ounce of discretion is a pound of learning.
- Planning is a continuous learning experience.

- A plan is blue print for taking action.
- Learning by doing. If I hear, I forget. If I see, I remember. If I do, I know.
- Work place is one of the most important institutions for providing human satisfaction.
- Survivability of any organization depends on its adaptability.
- The future is uncertain.
- An organization high on productivity is meeting to some degree, its goal attainments.
- Motivation may be defined as the degree to which individual motives are gratified.
- Rate of turnover, absenteeism and sick reports are common measures of motivation.
- Ego of knowledge without practical experience is a debilitated downfall of learning.
- Success is never an accident.
- Always praise in public and criticize in private.
- Role, functions and tasks of general management have been codified as—"Principles of Management".
- No one can discharge his duty without responsibilities.
- Manager should set the good examples through their actions and behaviors.
- Equal pay for equal work!
- Unnecessary turnover of employees is both the cause and effect of the bad management.
- Coordination is nothing but a mental attitude.
- Effective individuals are highly motivated one.
- High motivation and commitment helps to overcome frustrations, dejections and failures.
- Positive attitude, perceptual ability, cognitive flexibility and motivation are essential for creating orientation.
- Effective individual undertake several specialties.
- Coordination is one of the functions of leadership.
- Administrative personal must be compatible with each other.
- Continuous, on going, self evaluation is a means of quality assurance.
- Coordination is basic to practice of management at all levels.
- Emotion does play a part in negotiation session but guard against them.
- Delegation refers to operational authority only.
- Delegation is the most important parameter of managerial effectiveness.
- Organization is a dynamic concept.

- There is no single best leadership style.
- Group activity is not possible without communication.
- We can think four times faster than we can speak.
- Planning is looking forward and control is looking backward.
- Manager cannot have unlimited authority.
- Line organization is the backbone of the hierarchy.
- Functional authority is usually limited to the areas of how and sometimes when, but seldom to where, what or who.
- Well-trained and motivated workers do not need much supervision as others.
- A manager cannot do everything by himself.
- Unclear authority delegation is the most serious symptom of poor organization.
- Superior delegates authority not the responsibility.
- Multiple subordination must be avoided.
- Delegated authority must be commensurate with expected outcomes.
- A manager cannot delegate authority which he does not have.
- Employees should receive orders from one superior only.
- Order is a place for everything and everything in its place.
- Responsibility must be matched by authority.
- Understand employees, their needs, and aspirations and knit them together as a team.
- Planning cannot be delegated.
- Plans provide an opportunity for the organization to be proactive rather than reactive.
- Organization hierarchy refers to arrangement of individuals into series of superiors and subordinates.
- One of the pitfalls in problem identification is to miss the woods for the trees.
- It is impossible to plan for all the problems at all the time simultaneously.
- Short-term goals generally have a greater degree of specificity than long-term goals.
- A plan had no value if it remains only in the mind of planner.
- From the value judge angle, decision can be of two types—those that are expensive to change, and those that are not.
- Principal goal in decision making is to achieve maximum payoff at minimum cost.
- Right perception of decision-making process determines the success of decision making.

- In every organization, there should be a clear line of authority for everyone.
- Responsibility cannot be greater than the authority vested in a person.
- Manager cannot delegate all their authority completely.
- Centralization or decentralization is governed by policy, uniformity and size of the organization.
- One-way communication is usually not much effective.
- People often want more than money from a job.
- Communication is one of the forces for influencing staff direction.
- A good leader has to be a good listener.
- People want to be heard, to be taken seriously, to be understood.
- Where human relationships count in performance, it is hard to measure what is good, effective or efficient.
- One cannot know where the responsibility for deviations is, unless organization responsibility is clear and defined.
- For control process, organization structure is very important element.
- Implementation of any program always needs careful planning and dedicated person.
- Effective professional have positive attitude toward themselves, towards others and the system in which they work.
- Make a prioritized list of everything you need to do.
- Give the best to the recipients irrespective of the background.
- We may be small, but our goal is tall.
- Delegation of authority is not absolute and permanent.
- Autograph your work with excellence.
- Every work is a self-portrait of the person who done it.
- Always find profit from our mistakes.
- Our mistakes are our best masters.
- All business operations can be reduced to three words: People, product and profit.
- Time is the only resource which cannot be expanded.
- Be open to all criticism and comments.
- Remember, failure is a part of the human experience.
- Nobody is infallible.
- Nobody is always right all the time.
- To make a mistake is our own right.
- The only person who never makes a mistake is the man who does nothing.
- Be creative, initiative and innovative.

- An administrator who is not "fired with enthusiasm" should be fire, with enthusiasm.
- There is competition all around, there is place for all.
- Do not panic.
- Do not overestimate the qualities of your organization.
- If problem was not difficult, it will not be a problem.
- Competency comes from knowledge, skills and experience.
- Effective administration is a skill.
- Devotes sufficient time and energy for what is important.
- Urgent will anyway be got done.
- Always aim higher you will come up better.
- Never underestimate your power and capacity.
- Do not underestimate your problems.
- Have faith in yourself and in your organization.
- He who shoots at the sun will shoot higher than he who shoots at a tree.
- Give credit to your fellow workers.
- Use your authority sparingly and when clearly indicated.
- Do your homework carefully and regularly.
- Know everything about your organization.
- Distinguish between what is important and what is urgent.
- Meeting helps in the meeting of mind.
- Every meeting must have an aim and agenda.
- Delegation without authority is not delegation at all.
- Listen attentively and learn to disagree agreeably.
- Satisfaction an important aspect in negotiation.
- He who has patience can have what he will.
- Always take time to work out the implications.
- There can be no progress without change.
- To innovate means to introduce something new, to be creative.
- Imagination is the workshop of the mind.
- Our mind is compare to parachute; they function only when they are open.
- Those who think they can and done get new thing done.
- To be innovative, one has to be something of a dreamer and doer.
- If you wish to succeed, you must have a definite aim and purpose.
- Always anticipate the needs of your organization.
- Initiative is the pass-key that opens the door to the opportunity.
- Without accurate information, one cannot produce the desire changes.
- Purpose of delegation is to enable the administrator to concentrate on his own job.

- Delegation cannot be indiscriminate.
- Decision may be positive or negative.
- Decision may or may not lead to solution of the problem at the same time.
- Monitoring is concerned with day-to-day activities; evaluation is concerned with long-term assessment.
- Evaluation is the process of data collection and using the data to form judgment.
- Evaluation is an integral part of planning.
- Time is one of the greatest resources.
- Always carry with you a pocket diary.
- Learn to say "NO" graciously.
- If you have nothing to do, do not do it here.
- Do not allow others, who have nothing better to do, waste your precious time.
- Do not do yourself what someone else can do better.
- Do not waste time in unnecessary arguments, even if you win, you lose in goodwill.
- Do not brood over the past failure and mistakes.
- Let time serve you. Let it not be your master but your servant.
- A leader must not only be honest in his dealings, but he must also appear to be honest.
- Fear of failure can only result in failure.
- Do not be afraid of opposition.
- Decision making is the heart of all managerial function.
- A leader dreams things that never were and say why not!
- Leadership is doing right thing in the right manner at the right time as a matter of right.
- Delegation is ineffective without feedback and control.
- Enthusiasm is contagious. Let everyone catch it!
- Great achievements come with great sacrifice.
- Understand the needs of others and be sensitive to day-to-day behavior.
- Planning raises all the questions of what, why, where, when, who, and how as also how much and how many.
- Indians are said to be good in planning but poor in implementation.
- Do not rest until core problem is identified.
- Information is only a tool for better administration.
- Do not assume that what is known to you is known to everyone else.
- Effective communication is an essential catalyst for good performance.
- Equity may mean many things to many people.

- Decision making and problem solving is not the same thing.
- Quality control is not one time retrospective audit.
- Balance sheet is a snapshot picture of assets and liabilities on a particular date.
- Who knows best about individual's performance is an important issue in appraisal.
- Take care of your people.
- Technology is changing fast all the time.
- Communication is easier when there is mutual trust.
- Information is a source of power.
- Only constant feature in this world is change.
- An important requirement for innovation is learning from experience.
- Change is crucial and must for progress.
- Best communicator is the best manager.
- Anticipate the problem and try to solve the problem before.
- Do not go for unrealistic thing.
- Not to complain all the time but try to find out solution.
- Do not be liberal in such a way that damage the reputation of the organization.
- Be a quality assurance, not only focus on profit.
- Automation is the biggest business.
- As a manager, invite the newer technology all the time.
- Never entertain personnel conflict.
- Political nuisance is everywhere.
- Work according to laws, rules and regulation.
- Manager may not be an emotional.
- In case of conflict, take an expert opinion.
- Hidden agenda never dilute.
- Remember professional people are expert people.
- Goal setting itself a motivating factor.
- Million said the apple fell but only Newton was the one to ask—"Why".
- Delay is the financial disaster.
- Focus on why, where and how much excess money is spent.
- First step for one may be last step for another.
- Making money and spending it foolishly was completely meaningless.
- All difficulties in your life have a purpose.
- Be concerned that you do not offend, not that you are not offend.
- Always keep your thoughts on positive side.
- Retirement should mean, not a cessation of activity, but a change of activity with a more complete giving of your life to service.

- Your motives must be good if your work is to have good effects.
- In a conflict situation you must be thinking of a solution which is fair to all concerned.
- You cannot change anyone except yourself.
- There is always a way to do right!
- Always assume right attitude toward life.
- Overcome evil with good, falsehood with truth, and hatred with peace.
- An empty mind is devil's workshop.
- If you cannot fly, run. If you cannot run, walk. If you cannot walk, crawl.
- Whatever you do, keep moving toward your goal.
- Creative thinking is an art to cultivate, a skill to develop, a process to enjoy.
- Quality management program promote job satisfaction.
- No extra efforts are required to develop creative thinking other than to have a focused vision.
- *Five great Gurus are:* What, Why, Who, When and Where.
- Creative thinking is nothing but constructive thoughts that lead to productive outcome.
- Attitudinal change is complex, but not difficult.
- Management means getting things done through others.
- Everybody responsible means no body is responsible.
- You can gain an extra hour by daily to do list.
- Information explosion, global competition, total quality, and diversity are some of the harsh reality facing managers today.
- If you know how to manage men then rest of the things will be managed by themselves.
- The competition can copy your technology, but they cannot copy the creativity, knowledge, competency, and value of your committed workforce.
- Organization that do not change suffer from entrophy and soon become defunct.
- No organization can stand still and tread water for very long.
- Remember human capital cannot be replaced.
- What is important is to add life into years and not years into your life.
- If you spent yesterday in remaining gloomy over some mistake, do not spend today in regretting that gloom.
- How you spend your time is more important than how you spend your money.
- Money mistake can be corrected, but time is gone forever.
- The best use of time is to spend it after something that is everlasting.

- We need time to dream, time to remember, and time to reach the infinite.
- A man who dares to waste one hour of time has not discovered the value of life.
- A calendar does not care how you spend your time.
- You will never find time for anything. If you want time you must make it.
- To choose time is to save time.
- Spend less time worrying who is right and wrong and more time deciding what is right and wrong.
- The way you manage your time determines your destiny.
- Do not say you do not have enough time. You have the same numbers of hours per day as Mahatma Gandhiji, Mother Teresa, and Albert Einstein.
- If you keep waiting for just right time, you may never begin.
- Do not let your eyes moisten for the lost opportunity. Keep them clear so that you do not miss the upcoming opportunity.
- Not only strike while the iron is hot, but make it hot by striking.
- Do not waste your time waiting for inspiration. Begin and inspiration will find you.
- Do not delay acting on a good idea. Chances are, someone else has just thought of it too. Success comes to the one who acts first.
- It is better to change yourself to utilize the opportunity available to you than to change opportunity.
- Do your best every day and be free from all your grievances.
- Do not use time and words carelessly. Neither can be retrieved.
- Punctuality should be made not only a point of courtesy but also a point of conscience.
- Time is too slow for those who wait, too swift for those who fear, too long for those who grieve and too short for those who rejoice.
- Character is the result of two things—mental attitude and way we spend our time.
- How wonderful it is that nobody need wait a single moment before starting to improve the world.
- Best way to attract others is to keep yourself cool whenever they are hot at you.
- Skill with people is the most rewarding of all human talents.
- People are primarily interested in themselves, not in you.
- Understand people and their nature is the first step toward successful human relation.

- Take these four words out of your vocabulary—I, Me, My, and Mine.
- People would rather talk about themselves than about any other subjects.
- When talking to others, talk about them and get them talking about themselves.
- Never argue with anyone, even if you are right.
- More listening you do, the smarter you will become, the better you will be liked, and the better conversationalist you will be.
- Satisfied customers are the best advertisement.
- Everything in this world is done for a reason.
- Man does not live on bread alone!
- The man who cannot believe in himself cannot believe in anything else.
- Quality control and assessment is the integral part of management.
- Managers mainly carry out the functions of planning, organizing, staffing, leading and controlling.
- High quality is the best advertisement.
- Conflicts demand attention.
- Leader is a part of the group.
- Distinct from the group of and can influence the behavior of the group.
- Criticism should be made in absolute privacy.
- Demanding is a last resort measure.
- Always stand on your merits.
- A minimum of two persons are essential to form a management.
- Management is the activity of man who struggles for better living in the complex and competitive world.
- Nothing can be performed without planning.
- Management is must for every enterprise.
- Resources will remain merely as resources without management.
- Management meets the challenge of change.
- There are eight "M" in the business—Men, Money, Material, Machines, Methods, Motivation, Markets, and Management.
- Efficient management is the lifeboat of any developed business.
- Sleepless is one of the best investment you can make to make your life more productive and rewarding.
- Set aside one hour every morning for personal developmental matters.
- Starting the day off well is a powerful strategy for self-renewal.
- Quality management is a means of ensuring efficiency and effectiveness.
- Build a mystique around yourself.

- Empty your cup. A full cup cannot accept anything more. Similarly, a person who believes that he cannot learn anything else will stagnate quickly and not move to higher levels.
- A manager cannot delegate all of his authority.
- All individuals who have attained the highest of levels generally have cultivated the essential mental habit of optimism, without optimism, life loses its luster and hardships appear at every step.
- Laughter activates many beneficial chemicals within the body that place us into a very joyous state. Laughter also returns the body to a state of balance.
- Always spend some time with nature. Natural settings have a powerful effect on your senses which in turn will lead to a sense of renewal, refreshment and peacefulness.
- Set aside every Sunday evening for yourself and your family and be strongly disciplined with this habit.
- Become your spouse's number one supporter, the one who is always there supporting and fueling hopes and dreams. Develop together and march confidently through the world as army of two.
- To enhance your concentration and power of focus, count your steps when you walk. So many people allow their minds to be filled with mental chatter. All peak performers appreciate the power of a quiet clear mind which will concentrate steadily on all important tasks.
- Enhance your will power. You must first exercise it and then push before it gets stronger.
- Be careful about your reputation. Never do anything you would not be proud to tell your mother about. Have a fun always but temper it with common sense and prudence.
- Cultivate the art of walking half an hour after your dinner. Walks in natural settings are the very best. Walking is, perhaps, nature's ideal exercise.
- Never discuss your health, wealth and other personal matters with anyone outside your immediate family. Be very disciplined in this regard.
- Aromas have been proven to be effective means of entering a state of relaxation.
- Scents have a very noticeable effect on your mindsets and moods.
- Always remember the key principle that the quality of your life is the quality of your communication. This means the way you communicate with others and more importantly with yourself. What you focus on is what you get.

- A contented mind is a continual feast. Greed and material desires must be curbed to achieve lasting happiness and serenity. Be happy with what you have.
- Remember and use people's name when you talk to them.
- A person's name is a uniquely sweet sound to them.
- Get away from your rigid schedule which will provide a refreshing release and make you feel wonderful when you eventually return.
- You sow an action, you reap a habit. You sow a habit, you reap a character. You sow a character, you reap a destiny. Speak truth and measure your words wisely.
- Be humble, straight forward, and peaceful.
- Do not say you will do anything unless you will indeed do it.
- Be known as someone with a cool head, warm heart and great character. Your presence on this earth will long be remembered.
- Develop the essential habit of punctuality for it is most important for high success. Punctuality reflects discipline and proper regards for others. Without it, even the most sophisticated person appears slightly offensive.
- Every day, get away from the noise, the crowds and the rush and spend a few hours alone in peaceful introspection, deep reading or simple relaxation.
- Readers are leaders. Some top performers read a book a day.
- The more you know the less you fear.
- Drink a cup of warm water before a speech. You will be judged by the caliber of your communication skills.
- Never argue with person you work for—you will lose more than just the argument.
- Recognize the power of *mantras* and the repetition of positive, powerful words. Indian yogis have employed this technique for over 4000 years to live tranquil, productive and focused lives.
- Winners do the things that less developed people do not like doing even though they also might not enjoy doing them. This is what strength of character and courage is all about.
- Read the biographies of the world's leaders and learn from habits, inspirations and philosophies. Cultivate the important practice of active role modeling.
- Laugh at work and be known as a positive achiever.
- Keep well informed about current events, the latest books and populars trends. Many peak performers read five or six papers a day. You do not have to read every story of every paper. Know what to focus on.

- Four kinds of people:
  People who watch things happen,
  People to whom things happen,
  People who do not know what is happening and people who make things happen.
- Take chances, take smart risks and you will meet with success beyond your dreams.
- Each day, do two things that you do not like doing. This may be preparation of a report you have been putting off or shining your shoes. Your personal power will increase and your productivity will soar.
- Do not take personal development book as gospel. Read them and take whatever useful ideas you need. Every book has at least one tool or strategy of benefit.
- Pick five relationships that you desire to improve over the next 6 months. Write out the names of these people and under each name detail why you want to improve the relationship, how you plan to do so and in what time frame. This is simply another facet of goal setting.
- Coming together is beginning, keeping together is progress, and working together is success.
- Communication is the means by which change is affected, behaviors are modified and information is made productive.
- Evaluation is must to know the result of the training.

From Expert's Desks (FED)

To manage is to forecast and plan, to organize, to command, to co-ordinate and to control. **– Henry Fayol**

Management is doing things right; Leadership is doing the right things. **– Peter Drucker**

Management is the function of executive leadership anywhere. **– Ralph Davis**

Power is the probability that one acts within a social constraint to carry out his own will despite resistance. **– Max Weber**

An organization is a lengthened shadow of a man. **– Ralph Emerson**

Management is what a manager does! **– Louis Allan**

Management must manage! **– Harold S Geneen**

I call that man idle who might be better employed. **– Socrates**

Management is efficiency in climbing the ladder of success; Leadership determines whether the ladder is leaning against the right wall. **– Stephen Covey**

In that way imagination and intelligence enter into our existence in the part of servants of the primary instincts. **– Albert Einstein**

Management by objective works—if you know the objectives. 90% of the time you don't. **– Peter Drucker**

Management is defined for conceptual, theoretical, and analytical purposes as that process by which manager create, direct, maintain and operate purposive organization through systemic, coordinated cooperative human effort. **– Mc Farland**

Management is nothing more than motivating other people. **– Lee Iacocca**

Most of what we call management consists of making it difficult for people to get their work done. **– Peter Drucker**

Effective leadership is putting first things first. Effective management is discipline, carrying it out. **– Stephen Covey**

Management is the art of getting things done through and with an informally organized groups. **– Harold Koonts**

Wages are paid out of a predetermined fund of wealth which lay surplus with wealthy persons as a result of saving. This fund could be utilized for employing laborers for work. **– Adam Smith**

Management is about arranging and telling. Leadership is about nurturing and enhancing. **– Thomas J Peters**

If your actions inspire others to dream more, learn more, do more and become more, you are a leader. **– John Quincy Adams**

All of the great leaders have had one characteristic in common: It was the willingness to confront unequivocally the major anxiety of their people in their time. This, and not much else, is the essence of leadership.

– John Kenneth Galbraith

Struggle is the father of all things. It is not by the principles of humanity that man lives or is able to preserve himself above the animal world, but solely by means of the most brutal struggle. **– Adolf Hitler**

Good management consists in showing average people how to do the work of superior people. **– John D Rockefeller**

Management is that function of an enterprise which concern itself with direction and control of the various activities to attain business objectives. Management is essentially an executive functions, it deals with the active direction of the human efforts. **– William Spriegel**

Imagination is more important than intelligent. **– Albert Einstein**

Eliminate numerical quotas, including Management by Objectives.

– Edwards Deming

Management is an organ; organs can be described and defined only through their functions. **Peter Drucker**

The first rule of management is delegation. Don't try and do everything yourself because you can't. **– Anthea Turner**

The nearest analogy is in the human body. Personnel management is not the brain, the controller, not only just the limb, a member: not yet the blood streams, the energizing force, it is the nervous system. It is a line channel, not just a duct, and in some respect has automotive force. **– Aldrich**

Practice Golden-Rule 1 of Management in everything you do. Manage others the way you would like to be managed. **– Brian Tracy**

Money incentives alone not bring the desire motivation. Employees in an industry are not 'economic men' so much as they are 'ego men.' What they want, above all else, is credit for work done, interesting tasks, appreciation, approval and congenial relations with their employers and fellow-workers. These satisfactions they want even more than high wages or job security.

– Allen Port

Aim of argument or of discussion should not be victory but progress.

– Joseph Joubert

Management is not people; it is an activity like walking, reading. People who perform management can be designated as managers, members of management or executive leaders. **– Unknown**

The conventional definition of management is getting work done through people, but real management is developing people through work.

– Agha Hasan Abedi

A great profit without risk, experience without danger, and reward without hard work, is as impossible as it is to live without being born.

– AP Gouthey

Man is not the creature of circumstances; Circumstances are the creature of man. **– Benjamin Disrachi**

Being ignorant is not so much a shame as being unwilling to learn.

– Benjamin Franklin

Management manages by making decisions and by seeing that those decisions are implemented. **– Harold S Geneen**

Action is the product of the qualities inherent in nature.

– Bhagavad Gita

Apart from the humanitarian reasons, there are strong reasons why manager should take health and safety seriously because stress in manager is very dangerous. **– Bradford**

Effective management always means asking the right question.

– Robert Heller

The smaller the function, the greater the management.

– C Northcote Parkinson

This is the key to time management—to see the value of every moment.
– Menachem Mendel

The person who goes farthest is generally the one who is willing to do and dare. The sure thing boat never gets far from shore. **– Dale Carnegle**

The way forward for effective supervision is to maintain keep trust, be practice, and rational but not to police the workers. **– David Wimpress**

Management is not a matter of pressing a button, pulling a lever, issuing orders, scanning profit and loss statements, promulgating rules and regulations, rather it is power to determine what shall happen to the personalities and happiness of entire people, the power to shape the destiny of the nation and of all the nations which make up the world.
– Unknown

Natural abilities are like natural plants; they need pruning by study.
– Francis Bacon

A group of men who individually can do nothing, but as a group decide that nothing can be done. **– Fred Allen**

Power means the ability to get an individual or group to do something to get the person or group to change in some way. **– Fred Luthans**

To fail is not unworthy, since it implies that one had attempted something. **– George Clemenceau**

We will either find a way, or make one. **– Hannibal**

Picture yourself vividly as winning, and the alone will contribute immeasurably to success. **– Harry Emerson Fosdick**

Failure is the only opportunity to begin again more intelligently.
– Henry Ford

Every problem has in it the seeds of its own solution. If you don't have any problems, you don't get any seeds. **– Norman Vincent Peale**

Great things are not done by impulse, but by series of small things brought together. **– Vincent Van Gogh**

Good management is the art of making problems so interesting and their solutions so constructive that everyone wants to get to work and deal with them. **– Paul Hawken**

Each work has to pass through these stages—ridicule, opposition, and then acceptance. Those who think ahead of their time are sure to be misunderstood. **– Swami Vivekananda**

A lie can be half round the world before the truth has got its boots on. **– James Callaghan**

Singleness of purpose is one of the chief essential for success in life. **– John D Rockefeller**

The art of communication is the language of leadership. **– James Humes**

Only in men's imagination does every truth find an effective and undeniable existence. Imagination, not invention, is the supreme master of arts as of life. **– Joseph Conrad**

Yesterday is the cancelled cheque, tomorrow is a promissory note, today is the only cash you have so spend it wisely. **– Kay Lyons**

Your hearts know in silence the secrets of the days and the nights. **– Khalil Gibran**

Apply yourself. Get all the education you can, but then, by God, do something. Don't just stand there, make it happen. **– Lee Iacocca**

A man is the sum of his actions, of what he has done, of what he can do, nothing else. **– Mahatma Gandhiji**

Look at a day when you are supremely satisfied at the end. It's not a day when you lounge around doing nothing; it's when you have had everything to do, and you have done it. **– Margaret Thatcher**

The best job goes to the person who can get it done without passing the buck or coming back with excuses. **– Napoleon Hill**

Pictures help you to form the mental mold. **– Robert Collier**

Brings idea in and entertain them royally, for one of them may be king. **– Mark Van Doren**

Behavior study of human is looking into a deep well, how you can receive the best elixir of life from it. **– Pujya Motta**

A group of the unfit, appointed by the unwilling, to do the unnecessary. **– Stewart Harrol**

We are responsible for what we are, and whatever we wish ourselves to be, we have the power to make ourselves. If what we are now has been the result of our own past actions, it certainly follows that whatever we wish to be in future can be produced by our present actions; so we have to know how to act. **– Swami Vivekananda**

Success is relative. It is what we can make of the mess we have made of things. **– TS Eliot**

Where is the wisdom? We have lost in knowledge? Where is the knowledge we have lost in information. **– TS Eliot**

Decision making process can be analoged with a rolling stone that might hammer one's head or hang on the way hard if not handled properly. **– Tom Peters**

Sitting on a committee is like sitting on a commode. You make a lot of noise and finally drop the whole matter. **– Winston Churchill**

The word management, "Denotes a function but also the people who discharge it. It denotes a social position and rank but also a discipline and field of study. **– Peter Ducker**

When a management with a reputation for brilliance tackles a business with a reputation for bad economics, it is the reputation of the business that remains intact. **– Warren Buffett**

Fit no stereotypes. Don't chase the latest management fads. The situation dictates which approach best accomplishes the team's mission. **– Colin Powell**

Most of what we call management consists of making it difficult for people to get their work done. **– Peter Drucker**

Divorced from ethics, leadership is reduced to management and politics to mere technique. **– James Mac Gregor Burns**

Fit no stereotypes. Don't chase the latest management fads. The situation dictates which approach best accomplishes the team's mission. **– Colin Powell**

If a sufficient number of management layers are superimposed on top of each other, it can be assured that disaster is not left to chance. **– Norman Ralph Augustine**

If I had learned more about business ahead of time, I would have been shaped into believing that it was only about finances and quality management. **– Anita Roddick**

Index investing out performs active management year after year. **– Jim Rogers**

It is not enough to have great qualities; we should also have the management of them. **– Francois de La Rochefoucauld**

It was to do with information management. The intention was to dramatize it. **– Hans Blix**

It's not just buying the company. Sure, we picked the right companies, and we picked the right management and, most importantly, we've given them the right incentive to perform. **– Henry Kravis**

Lots of folks confuse bad management with destiny. **– Kin Hubbard**

Management doesn't really have any problem at all with firing people.

It's a powerful idea that, If I'm not happy, I'll quit. I'll try something else! **– Ron Livingston**

Management must speak with one voice. When it doesn't management itself becomes a peripheral opponent to the team's mission. **– Pat Riley**

Leaders establish the vision for the future and set the strategy for getting there; they cause change. They motivate and inspire others to go in the right direction and they, along with everyone else, sacrifice to get there. **– John Kotter**

No business in the world has ever made more money with poorer management. **– Bill Terry**

Security is always going to be a cat and mouse game because there'll be people out there that are hunting for the zero day award, you have people that don't have configuration management, don't have vulnerability management, don't have patch management. **– Kevin Mitnick**

So much of what we call management consists in making it difficult for people to work. **– Peter Drucker**

The art of effective listening is essential to clear communication, and clear communication is necessary to management success. **– James Cash Penney**

The budget evolved from a management tool into an obstacle to management. **– Charles Edwards**

The Democrats seem to be basically nicer people, but they have demonstrated time and again that they have the management skills of celery. **– Dave Barry**

The difference between management and administration (which is what bureaucrats used to do exclusively) is the difference between choice and rigidity. **– Robert Heller**

First myth of management is that it exists. Second myth of management is that success equals skill. **– Robert Heller**

The kind of people I look for to fill top management spots are the eager beavers, the mavericks. These are the guys who try to do more than they're expected to do—they always reach. **– Lee Iacocca**

Leadership is getting people to work for you when they are not obligated. **– Fred Smith**

The leader will be a person with the management skills to coordinate the activities of the team, and to assure that the team remains faithful to the objectives of the incoming President. **– Richard V Allen**

The outstanding people realized that the job involved more than just writing a good strategic plan. It was also important that top management should understand the plan and be prepared to adopt it. **– David C McClelland**

The relationship between talent and management is uneasy, at best. **– Jessica Savitch**

The secret to winning is constant, consistent management. **– Tom Landry**

The time draws near, when a radical change must take place for the whole world in the management of diplomacy. **– Lajos Kossuth**

The first responsibility of a leader is to define reality. The last is to say thank you. In between, the leader is a servant. **– Max De Pree**

There is no single development, in either technology or management technique, which by itself promises even one order of—magnitude improvement within a decade in productivity, in reliability, in simplicity. **– Frederick P Brooks, Jr**

This constitution recognises the need for social dialogue involving labor and management; it involves trade unions in the decision making process; it has a social vision founded on social dialogue. **– Jean-Pierre Raffarin**

To sin by silence when they should protest makes cowards of men.
– Abraham Lincon

This legislation confronts the human truth that the need for clean water knows no borders, and proper management and intervention can be a currency for peace and international cooperation. **– Bill Frist**

Time management is a big part of the director's job. **– Debbie Allen**

We got great ratings and fan interest, and that's what management wanted.
– Trish Stratus

Good managers play checkers. Great managers play chess.
– Marcus Buckingham

Leadership is the activity of influencing people to cooperate toward some goal which they come to find desirable. **– Ordway Tead**

We have problems with our physical security, operational security through to management. **– Kevin Mitnick**

We need what I have often called an ecological approach to the management of these resources and we do not have that now. We have the inertia of past habits, unsustainable habits. **– Maurice Strong**

We ought to have more women in various management positions, because women are the ones who decide almost everything in the home.
– Ingvar Kamprad

We're just delighted that management has come around to my way of thinking. **– Paula Zahn**

People ask the difference between a leader and a boss. The leader leads, and the boss drives. **– Theodore Roosevelt**

Leadership is not so much about technique and methods as it is about opening the heart. Leadership is about inspiration—of oneself and of others. Great leadership is about human experiences, not processes. Leadership is not a formula or a program, it is a human activity that comes from the heart and considers the hearts of others. It is an attitude, not a routine.
– Lance Secretan

We've got a low turnover management group and executive group who've grown up in the business. **– Fred L Turner**

Leadership is a serving relationship that has the effect of facilitating human development. **– Ted Ward**

When you're buying real growth and want real performance, you buy excellent management and good products and you diversify across industry sectors. **– Robert Morse**

Leadership cannot really be taught. It can only be learned. **– Harold Geneen**

When a management with a reputation for brilliance tackles a business with a reputation for bad economics, it is the reputation of the business that remains intact. **– Warren Buffett**

Reduce the layers of management. They put distance between the top of an organization and the customers. **– Donald Rumsfeld**

Developing excellent communication skills is absolutely essential to effective leadership. The leader must be able to share knowledge and ideas to transmit a sense of urgency and enthusiasm to others. If a leader can't get a message across clearly and motivate others to act on it, then having a message doesn't even matter. **– Gilbert Amelio**

Leadership is intentional influence. **– Michael McKinney**

Motivation is everything. You can do the work of two people, but you can't be two people. Instead, you have to inspire the next guy down the line and get him to inspire his people. **– Lee Iacocca**

He who has never learned to obey cannot be a good commander. **– Aristotle**

The great thing is to know when to speak and when to keep quiet. **– Seneca the Younger**

When customers complain, business owners and managers ought to get excited about it. The complaining customer represents a huge opportunity for more business. **– Zig Ziglar**

If you pick the right people and give them the opportunity to spread their wings—and put compensation as a carrier behind it—you almost don't have to manage them. **– Jack Welch**

Never try to teach a pig to sing; it wastes your time and it annoys the pig.
– Paul Dickson

Because a thing seems difficult for you, do not think it impossible for anyone to accomplish. **– Marcus Aurelius**

When hiring key employees, there are only two qualities to look for: judgement and taste. Almost everything else can be bought by the yard.
– John W Gardner

Good management is the art of making problems so interesting and their solutions so constructive that everyone wants to get to work and deal with them. **– Paul Hawken**

Control is not leadership; management is not leadership; leadership is leadership. If you seek to lead, invest at least 50% of your time in leading yourself—your own purpose, ethics, principles, motivation, conduct. Invest at least 20% leading those with authority over you and 15% leading your peers. **– Dee Hock**

Knowing is not enough, we must apply! Willing is not enough, we must do! **– Goethe**

If you can dream it, you can do it. **– Walt Disney**

It is better to keep your mouth closed and let people think you are a fool than to open it and remove all doubt. **– Mark Twain**

The most efficient way to produce anything is to bring together under one management as many as possible of the activities needed to turn out the product. **– Peter Drucker**

To lead people, walk beside them ... As for the best leaders, the people do not notice their existence. The next best, the people honor and praise. The next, the people fear; and the next, the people hate ... When the best leader's work is done the people say, 'We did it ourselves! **– Lao-tsu**

No institution can possibly survive if it needs geniuses or supermen to manage it. It must be organized in such a way as to be able to get along under a leadership composed of average human beings. **– Peter Drucker**

Always mistrust a subordinate who never finds fault with his superior.
– John Churton Collins

Tell me and I'll forget. Show me and I may remember. Involve me and I'll understand. **– Socrates**

We are what we repeatedly do. Excellence, therefore, is not an act but a habit. **– Aristotle**

Experience is the child of thought, and thought is the child of action. **– Benjamin Disraeli**

Nothing great was ever achieved without enthusiasm. **– Ralph Waldo Emerson**

The ability to concentrate and to use your time well is everything if you want to succeed in business—or almost anywhere else for that matter. **– Lee Iacocca**

The three most important words for a successful relationship are: communication, communication, and communication. **– Anonymous**

It is not enough to take steps which may someday lead to a goal; each step must be itself a goal and a step likewise. **– Johann Wolfgang von Goethe**

To do great things is difficult; but to command great things is more difficult. **– Friedrich Nietzsche**

The first ingredient in conversation is truth: the next good sense; the third, good humor; and the fourth wit. **– Sir William Temple**

Surround yourself with the best people you can find, delegate authority, and don't interfere as long as the policy you've decided upon is being carried out. **– Ronald Reagan**

Focus on a few key objectives ... I only have three things to do. I have to choose the right people, allocate the right number of dollars, and transmit ideas from one division to another with the speed of light. So I'm really in the business of being the gatekeeper and the transmitter of ideas. **– Jack Welch**

Leadership is the ability to establish standards and manage a creative climate where people are self-motivated toward the mastery of long term constructive goals, in a participatory environment of mutual respect, compatible with personal values. **– Mike Vance**

Motivation is the art of getting people to do what you want them to do because they want to do it. **– Dwight Eisenhower**

Opportunity is missed by most people because it comes dressed in overalls and looks like work. **– Thomas Edison**

There is only one valid definition of business purpose: To create a customer. **– Peter Drucker**

Health Quotations

Health is a state of complete physical, mental and social well-being, and not merely the absence of disease or infirmity.

– World Health Organization

Webster's dictionary denotes health as 'a condition of being sound in body, spirit, especially freedom from physical illness, disease or pain.'

Oxford dictionary defines it as 'soundness of body or mind, that condition in which its functions are duly and effectively discharged.'

Cambridge International dictionary states 'Health as a conditional body and degree to which it is free from illness or state of well-being.'

Chambers 21st dictionary defines it as 'a state of physical, mental and social well-being accompanied by freedom from illness or pain.'

The International Covenant on Economic, Social, and Cultural Rights (ICESCR) recognize that health is central to the dignity of the person and the state's commitment to health of the population as a fundamental human right.

Let food be thy medicine, thy medicine shall be thy food. **– Hippocrates**

New philosophy of health is:

Health is a fundamental right.

Health is essence of productive life.

Health is an intersectoral.

Health is integral part of development.

Health is concept of quality of life.

Health is worldwide social goal.

A Short History of Medicine:

2000 BC: "Here, eat this root."

1000 BC: "That root is heathen, say this prayer."

1850 AD: "That prayer is superstition, drink this potion."

1940 AD "That potion is snake oil, swallow this pill."

1985 AD: "That pill is ineffective, take this antibiotic."

2000 AD: "That antibiotic is artificial. Here, eat this root."

– Author Unknown

From the bitterness of disease man learns the sweetness of health.
– Catalan Proverb

When diet is wrong medicine is of no use.
When diet is correct medicine is of no need. **– Ayurvedic Proverb**

An imaginary ailment is worse than a disease. **– Yiddish Proverb**

He whose doshas (laws of nature at work in the body) are in balance, whose appetite is good, whose tissues are functioning normally, whose wastes are in balance, and whose Self, mind, and senses remain full of bliss, is called a healthy person. ***– Sushruta Samhita***

Leave your drugs in the chemist's pot, if you can heal the patient with food. **– Hippocrates**

There are lots of people in this world who spend so much time watching their health that they haven't the time to enjoy it. **– Josh Billings**

The greatest wealth is health. **– Virgil**

Only one rule in medical ethics need concern you—that action on your part which best conserves the interests of your patient. **– Martin H Fischer**

The highest ideal of cure is the rapid, gentle and permanent restoration of health by the most trustworthy and least harmful way.
– Samuel Hahnemann

The scientific truth may be put quite briefly; eat moderately, having an ordinary mixed diet, and don't worry. **– Robert Hutchison, 1932**

The mind has great influence over the body, and maladies often have their origin there. **– Moliere**

Surgeons must be very careful when they take the knife! Underneath their fine incisions stirs the Culprit - Life! **– Emily Dickinson**

The doctor of the future will give no medicine but will interest his patients in the care of the human frame, in diet and in the cause and prevention of disease. **– Thomas Edison**

Only freedom from prejudice and tireless zeal avail for the most holy of the endeavours of mankind, the practice of the true art of healing.
– Samuel Hahnemann

The best six doctors anywhere and no one can deny it
Are sunshine, water, rest, fresh air, exercise and diet.
These six will gladly you attend
If only you are willing
Your mind they'll ease
Your will they'll mend and charge you not a shilling.
– Nursery rhyme quoted by Wayne Fields, What the River Knows, 1990

A wise man ought to realize that health is his most valuable possession. **– Hippocrates**

I reckon being ill as one of the great pleasures of life, provided one is not too ill and is not obliged to work till one is better. **– Samuel Butler**

Health is a large word. It embraces not the body only, but the mind and spirit as well;... and not today's pain or pleasure alone, but the whole being and outlook of a man. **– James H West**

It is more important to know what sort of person has a disease than to know what sort of disease a person has. **– Hippocrates**

Life expectancy would grow by leaps and bounds, if green vegetables smelled as good as bacon. **– Doug Larson**

God and the Doctor we alike adore but only when in danger, not before; The danger o'er, both are alike requited, God is forgotten, and the Doctor slighted. **– Robert Owen**

So many people spend their health-gaining wealth, and then have to spend their wealth to regain their health. **– AJ Reb Materi, Our Family**

The art of healing comes from nature and not from the physician. Therefore, the physician must start from nature with an open mind. **– Paracelsus**

Medicine is a collection of uncertain prescriptions, the results of which taken collectively, are more fatal than useful to mankind. Water, air and cleanliness are the chief articles in my pharmacopeia. **– Napoleon Bonaparte**

The power of love to change bodies is legendary, built into folklore, common sense, and everyday experience. Love moves the flesh, it pushes matter around.... Throughout history, "tender loving care" has uniformly been recognized as a valuable element in healing. **– Larry Dossey**

Eat right, exercise regularly, die anyway. **– Author Unknown**

Health nuts are going to feel stupid someday, lying in hospitals dying of nothing. **– Redd Foxx**

The competent physician, before he attempts to give medicine to the patient, makes himself acquainted not only with the disease, but also with the habits and constitution of the sick man. **– Cicero**

As a people, we have become obsessed with health. There is something fundamentally, radically unhealthy about all this. We do not seem to be seeking more exuberance in living as much as staving off failure, putting off dying. We have lost all confidence in the human body. **– Lewis Thomas**

The fact that your patient gets well does not prove that your diagnosis was correct. **– Samuel J Meltzer**

In order to change we must be sick and tired of being sick and tired. **– Author Unknown**

He who takes medicine and neglects to diet wastes the skill of his doctors. **– Chinese Proverb**

When health is absent, Wisdom cannot reveal itself,
Art cannot become manifest, Strength cannot be exerted,
Wealth is useless and Reason is powerless. **– Herophilies, 300 BC**

Be careful about reading health books. You may die of a misprint. **– Mark Twain**

Physical ills are the taxes laid upon this wretched life; some are taxed higher, and some lower, but all pay something. **– Lord Chesterfield**

Drugs are not always necessary. Belief in recovery always is. **– Norman Cousins**

If the pain wanders, do not waste your time with doctors. **– Mignon McLaughlin**

The... patient should be made to understand that he or she must take charge of his own life. Don't take your body to the doctor as if he were a repair shop. **– Quentin Regestein**

Sickness comes on horseback but departs on foot. **– Dutch Proverb**

When you treat a disease, first treat the mind. **– Chen Jen**

Diseases of the soul are more dangerous and more numerous than those of the body.

– Cicero

If you have health, you probably will be happy, and if you have health and happiness, you have all the wealth you need, even if it is not all you want.

– Elbert Hubbard

People who are always taking care of their health are like misers who are hoarding a treasure which they have never spirit enough to enjoy.

– Laurence Sterne

To feel keenly the poetry of a morning's roses, one has to have just escaped from the claws of this vulture which we call sickness.

– Henri Frederic Amiel

A good laugh and a long sleep are the best cures in the doctor's book.

– Irish Proverb

Fresh air impoverishes the doctor.

– Danish Proverb

There are two things in life that a sage must preserve at every sacrifice, the coats of his stomach and the enamel of his teeth. Some evils admit of consolations, but there are no comforters for dyspepsia and the toothache.

– Henry Lytton Bulwer

The longer I live the less confidence I have in drugs and the greater is my confidence in the regulation and administration of diet and regimen.

– John Redman Coxe

The I in illness is isolation and the crucial letters in wellness are we.

– Author unknown

The best physician is one who knows the worthlessness of most medicines.

– Benjamin Franklin

No Illness which can be treated by the diet should be treated by any other means.

– Moses Maimonides

In minds crammed with thoughts, organs clogged with toxins, and bodies stiffened with neglect, there is just no space for anything else.

– Alison Rose Levy

The field of Western medicine has become literally nothing but medicine. Doctors are on their way out, to be replaced by self-serve pharmaceutical vending machines.

– Grey Livingston

In the nineteenth century, men lost their fear of God and acquired a fear of microbes. **– Author Unknown**

The sound body is the product of the sound mind.– **George Bernard Shaw**

Men that look no further than their outsides, think health an appurtenance to life, and quarrel with their constitutions for being sick; but I that have examined the parts of man, and know upon what tender filaments that fabric hangs, do wonder that we are not always so; and considering the thousand doors that lead to death, do thank God that we can die but once. **– Thomas Browne**

When it comes to eating right and exercising, there is no "I'll start tomorrow." Tomorrow is disease. **– Terri Guillemets**

What some call health, if purchased by perpetual anxiety about diet, isn't much better than tedious disease. **– George Dennison Prentice**

Illness is the most heeded of doctors: To goodness and wisdom we only make promises; pain we obey. **– Marcel Proust**

My own prescription for health is less paperwork and more running barefoot through the grass. **– Terri Guillemets**

We drink one another's health and spoil our own. **– Jerome K Jerome**

In a disordered mind, as in a disordered body, soundness of health is impossible. **– Cicero**

Health is a state of complete harmony of the body, mind and spirit. When one is free from physical disabilities and mental distractions, the gates of the soul open. **– BKS Iyengar**

Medicines heals doubts as well as diseases. **– Karl Marx**

Sickness is the vengeance of nature for the violation of her laws.
– Charles Simmons

The appearance of a disease is swift as an arrow; its disappearance slow, like a thread. **– Chinese Proverb**

It's the mind that makes the body rich. **– Shakespeare**

Anyone who believes that anything can be suited to everyone is a great fool, because medicine is practiced not on mankind in general, but on every individual in particular. **– Henri de Mondeville**

When a lot of remedies are suggested for a disease, that means it cannot be cured. **– Anton Chekhov**

Health is like munny, we never have a true idea of its value until we lose it. **– Josh Billings**

A healthy body and soul come from an unencumbered mind and body. **– Ymber Delecto**

Adam and Eve ate the first vitamins, including the package. **– ER Squibb**

Our body is a machine for living. It is organized for that, it is its nature. Let life go on in it unhindered and let it defend itself, it will do more than if you paralyze it by encumbering it with remedies. **– Leo Tolstoy**

Gold that buys health can never be ill spent. **– Thomas Dekker**

Disease is somatic; the suffering from it, psychic. **– Martin H Fischer**

Most over-the-counter and almost all prescribed drug treatments merely mask symptoms or control health problems or in some way alter the way organs or systems such as the circulatory system work. Drugs almost never deal with the reasons why these problems exist, while they frequently create new health problems as side effects of their activities. **– John R Lee**

Health of body and mind is a great blessing, if we can bear it. **– John Henry**

There are six components of wellness: Proper weight and diet, proper exercise, breaking the smoking habit, control of alcohol, stress management and periodic exams. **– Kenneth H Cooper**

Diseases crucify the soul of man, attenuate our bodies, dry them, wither them, rivel them up like old apples, make them as so many Anatomies. **– Robert Burton, The Anatomy of Melancholy**

A healthy body is the guest-chamber of the soul; a sick, its prison. **– Francis Bacon**

Hear your heart. Heart your health. **– Faith Seehill**

Preserving the health by too strict a regimen is a wearisome malady. **– François Duc de la Rochefoucauld**

If man thinks about his physical or moral state he usually discovers that he is ill. **– Johann Wolfgang von**

It's bizarre that the produce manager is more important to my children's health than the pediatrician. **– Meryl Streep**

Just because you're not sick doesn't mean you're healthy. **– Author Unknown**

Every man's disease is his personal property. **– Alonzo Clark**

Know, then, whatever cheerful and serene supports the mind supports the body too. **– John Armstrong**

When an illness knocks you on your ass, you should stay and relax for a while before trying to get back up. **– Terri Guillemets**

A bad cold wouldn't be so annoying if it weren't for the advice of our friends. **– Kin Hubbard**

Men make use of their illnesses at least as much as they are made use of by them. **– Aldous Huxley**

The greatest discovery of any generation is that human beings can alter their lives by altering the attitudes of their minds. **– Albert Schweitzer**

If you don't take care of yourself, the undertaker will overtake that responsibility for you. **– Carrie Latet**

The most important thing in illness is never to lose heart. **– Nikolai Lenin**

The part can never be well unless the whole is well. **– Plato**

If by gaining knowledge we destroy our health, we labour for a thing that will be useless in our hands. **– John Locke**

To avoid sickness eat less; to prolong life worry less. **– Chu Hui Weng**

When the headaches, all the body is the worse. **– English Proverb**

Healthy people are invalids who don't know it. **– Jules Romains, Dr Knock**

If your body's not right, the rest of your day will go all wrong. Take care of yourself. **– Terri Guillemets**

After these two, Dr Diet and Dr Quiet, Dr Merriman is requisite to preserve health. **– James Howell**

When a man is ill his very goodness is sickly. **– Friedrich Nietzsche**

The deviation of man from the state in which he was originally placed by nature seems to have proved to him a prolific source of disease.

– Edward Jenner

There is something in sickness that breaks down the pride of manhood.

– Charles Dickens

Bacteria keeps us from heaven and puts us there. **– Martin H Fischer**

Health and cheerfulness naturally beget each other. **– Joseph Addison**

It is a lot harder to keep people well than it is to just get them over a sickness. **– DeForest Clinton Jarvis**

Life is not merely to be alive, but to be well. **– Marcus Valerius Martial**

Confidence and hope do more good than physic. **– Galen**

Live in rooms full of light, avoid heavy food, and be moderate in the drinking of wine
Change surroundings and take long journeys
Take massage, baths, exercise, and gymnastics
Fight insomnia with gentle rocking or the sound of running water
Strictly avoid frightening ideas
Indulge in cheerful conversation and amusements
Listen to music. **– A Cornelius Celsus**

My inner advisor is dying to heal me. **– Astrid Alauda**

Everyone who is born holds dual citizenship, in the kingdom of the well and in the kingdom of the sick. Although we all prefer to use only the good passport, sooner or later each of us is obliged, at least for a spell, to identify ourselves as citizens of that other place.

– Susan Sontag, Illness as Metaphor

Half the modern drugs could well be thrown out the window, except that the birds might eat them. **– Martin H Fischer**

How sickness enlarges the dimension of a man's self to himself!

– Charles Lamb, Last Essays of Elia

Doctors are always working to preserve our health and cooks to destroy it, but the latter are the more often successful. **– Denis Diderot**

Sickness is poor-spirited, and cannot serve anyone; it must husband its resources to live. But health or fullness answers its own ends, and has to spare, runs over, and inundates the neighborhoods and creeks of other men's necessities. **– Ralph Waldo Emerson**

If you wish to keep as well as possible, the less you think about your health the better. **– Oliver Wendell**

First need in the reform of hospital management? That's easy! The death of all dietitians, and the resurrection of a French chef. **– Martin H Fischer**

In the face of such overwhelming statistical possibilities hypochondria has always seems to me to be the only rational position to take on life.
– John Diamond

He who has health has hope; and he who has hope has everything.
– Arabic Proverb

A bodily disease, which we look upon as whole and entire within itself, may, after all, be but a symptom of some ailment in the spiritual part.
– Nathaniel Hawthorne, The Scarlet Letter

Happiness lies, first of all, in health. **– George William Curtis**

The trouble with always trying to preserve the health of the body is that it is so difficult to do without destroying the health of the mind.
– GK Chesterton

If you start to think about your physical or moral condition, you usually find that you are sick. **– Johann Wolfgang von Goethe**

If you do everything you should do, and do not do anything you should not do, you will, according to the best available statistics, live exactly eighteen hours longer than you would otherwise. **– Logain Clendening**

It's no longer a question of staying healthy. It's a question of finding a sickness you like. **– Jackie Mason**

Health is merely the slowest way someone can die. **– Author Unknown**

May you live as long as you are fit to live, but no longer! or, may you rather die before you cease to be fit to live than after!
– Philip Dormer Stanhope

What linguistic genius set up the sneeze and wheeze
To rhyme so very perfectly with the word for allergies? – **Charlie N Abbers**

Those obsessed with health are not healthy; the first requisite of good health is a certain calculated carelessness about oneself. – **Sydney J Harris**

Nothing is more fatal to Health, than an over Care of it.
– **Benjamin Franklin**

The only way to keep your health is to eat what you don't want, drink what you don't like, and do what you'd druther not. – **Mark Twain**

In nothing do men more nearly approach the gods than in giving health to men. – **Cicero**

My doctor is nice; every time I see him, I'm ashamed of what I think of doctors in general. – **Mignon McLaughlin**

The greatest mistake in the treatment of diseases is that there are physicians for the body and physicians for the soul, although the two cannot be separated. – **Plato**

Body and soul cannot be separated for purposes of treatment, for they are one and indivisible. Sick minds must be healed as well as sick bodies.
– **C Jeff Miller**

In the sick room, ten cents' worth of human understanding equals ten dollars' worth of medical science. – **Martin H Fischer**

It is a mathematical fact that fifty percent of all doctors graduate in the bottom half of their class. – **Author Unknown**

Restore a man to his health, his purse lies open to thee. – **Robert Burton**

Being in control of your life and having realistic expectations about your day-to-day challenges are the keys to stress management, which is perhaps the most important ingredient to living a happy, healthy and rewarding life. – **Marilu Henner**

A hospital should also have a recovery room adjoining the cashier's office. – **Francis O'Walsh**

Did God who gave us flowers and trees, also provide the allergies?
– **EY Harburg**

It is a wise mans part, rather to avoid sickness, than to wishe for medicines. – **Thomas More**

You have a cough? Go home tonight, eat a whole box of Ex-Lax—tomorrow you'll be afraid to cough. **– Pearl Williams**

To array a man's will against his sickness is the supreme art of medicine. **– Henry Ward Beecher**

A doctor whose breath smells has no right to medical opinion. **– Martin H Fischer**

It is a good thing for a physician to have prematurely grey hair and itching piles. The first makes him appear to know more than he does, and the second gives him an expression of concern which the patient interprets as being on his behalf. **– A Benson Cannon**

A doctor who cannot take a good history and a patient who cannot give one are in danger of giving and receiving bad treatment. **– Author Unknown**

One thousand Americans stop smoking every day—by dying. **– Author Unknown**

A hypochondriac is one who has a pill for everything except what ails him. **– Mignon McLaughlin**

The art of medicine consists in amusing the patient while nature cures the disease. **– Voltaire**

A doctor must work eighteen hours a day and seven days a week. If you cannot console yourself to this, get out of the profession. **– Martin H Fischer**

It is sometimes as dangerous to be run into by a microbe as by a trolley car. **– JJ Walsh**

Every disease is a physician. **– Irish Proverb**

God heales, and the Physician hath the thankes. **– George Herbert, Outlandish Proverbs**

If the whole materia medica could be sunk to the bottom of the sea, it would be all the better for mankind and all the worse for the fishes. **– Oliver Wendell**

There is no curing a sick man who believes himself to be in health. **– Henri Amiel**

Doctors think a lot of patients are cured who have simply quit in disgust.
– Don Herold

The only equipment lack in the modern hospital? Somebody to meet you at the entrance with a handshake! **– Martin H Fischer**

The worst thing about medicine is that one kind makes another necessary. **– Elbert Hubbard**

When you are called to a sick man, be sure you know what the matter is—if you do not know, nature can do a great deal better than you can guess.
– Nicholas de Belleville

Poisons and medicine are oftentimes the same substance given with different intents. **– Peter Mere Latham**

Symptoms, then are in reality nothing but the cry from suffering organs.
– Jean Martin

Diagnosis is not the end, but the beginning of practice.
– Martin H Fischer

The physician should look upon the patient as a besieged city and try to rescue him with every means that art and science place at his command.
– Alexander of Tralles

Physicians and politicians resemble one another in this respect, that some defend the constitution and others destroy it. **– Author Unknown**

A smart mother makes often a better diagnosis than a poor doctor.
– August Bier

When fate arrives the physician becomes a fool. **– Arabic Proverb**

Medicines are not meat to live by. **– German Proverb**

Treat the patient, not the X-ray. **– James M Hunter**

Financial ruin from medical bills is almost exclusively an American disease. **– Roul Turley**

The hospital is the only proper College in which to rear a true disciple of Aesculapius. **– John Abernethy**

A man who cannot work without his hypodermic needle is a poor doctor. The amount of narcotic you use is inversely proportional to your skill.
– Martin H Fischer

Better to hunt in fields, for health unbought, Than fee the doctor for a nauseous draught,

The wise, for cure, on exercise depend; God never made his work for man to mend. **– John Dryden**

Medicine is the only profession that labours incessantly to destroy the reason for its own existence. **– James Bryce**

It is not a case we are treating; it is a living, palpitating, alas, too often suffering fellow creature. **– John Brown**

The patient does not care about your science; what he wants to know is, can you cure him? **– Martin H Fischer**

Developments in medical technology have long been confined to procedural or pharmaceutical advances, while neglecting a most basic and essential component of medicine: patient information management.
– John Doolittle

A physician is obligated to consider more than a diseased organ, more even than the whole man—he must view the man in his world.
– Harvey Cushing

Medicine sometimes snatches away health, sometimes gives it.
– Ovid, Tristia

As it takes two to make a quarrel, so it takes two to make a disease, the microbe and its host. **– Charles V Chapin**

Disease is war with the laws of our being, and all war, as a great general has said, is hell. **– Lewis G Janes**

Until a physician has killed one or two he is not a physician.
– *Kashmiri* Proverb

No man is a good doctor who has never been sick himself.
– Chinese Proverb

To me the ideal doctor would be a man endowed with profound knowledge of life and of the soul, intuitively divining any suffering or disorder of whatever kind, and restoring peace by his mere presence. **– Henri Amiel**

Medicinal discovery, It moves in mighty leaps, It leapt straight past the common cold and gives it us for keeps. **– Pam Ayres**

When you no longer know what headache, heartache, or stomachache means without cistern punctures, electrocardiograms and six X-ray plates, you are slipping. **– Martin H Fischer**

It is easy to get a thousand prescriptions but hard to get one single remedy. **– Chinese Proverb**

Never forget that it is not pneumonia, but a pneumonic man who is your patient. **– William Withey Gull**

It is said to be the manner of hypochondriacs to change often their physician. **– William Cullen**

The road to medical knowledge is through the pathological museum and not through an apothecary's shop. **– William Withey Gull**

A half doctor near is better than a whole one far away. **– German Proverb**

No doctor is better than three. **– German Proverb**

Man may be the captain of his fate, but is also the victim of his blood sugar. **– Wilfrid G Oakley**

Faith and knowledge lean largely upon each other in the practice of medicine. **– Peter Mere Latham**

Each patient ought to feel somewhat the better after the physician's visit, irrespective of the nature of the illness. **– Warfield Theobald Longcope**

Who ever thought up the word "Mammogram?" Every time I hear it, I think I'm supposed to put my breast in an envelope and send it to someone. **– Jan King**

Never go to a doctor whose office plants have died. **– Erma Bombeck**

You may know the intractability of a disease by its long list of remedies. **– Alonzo Clark**

Here's good advice for practice: Go into partnership with nature; she does more than half the work and asks none of the fee. **– Martin H Fischer**

Varicose veins are the result of an improper selection of grandparents. **– William Osler**

If you are too smart to pay the doctor, you had better be too smart to get ill. **– African Proverb**

Symptoms are the body's mother tongue; signs are in a foreign language.
– John Brown

Oh the powers of nature. She knows what we need, and the doctors know nothing.
– Benvenuto Cellini

So many come to the sickroom thinking of themselves as men of science fighting disease and not as healers with a little knowledge helping nature to get a sick man well.
– Auckland Geddes

Where a man feels pain he lays his hand. **– Dutch Proverb**

The doctor is often more to be feared than the disease. **– French Proverb**

Despite all our toil and progress, the art of medicine still falls somewhere between trout casting and spook writing.
– Ben Hecht, Miracle of the Fifteen Murderers

The Lord hath created medicines out of the earth; and he that is wise will not abhor them.
– Ecclesiasticus

A drug is that substance which, when injected into a rat, will produce a scientific report.
– Unknown

Cancer is a word, not a sentence. **– John Diamond**

The medicalization of early diagnosis not only hampers and discourages preventative healthcare but it also trains the patient-to-be to function in the meantime as an acolyte to his doctor. He learns to depend on the physician in sickness and in health. He turns into a life-long patient. **– Ivan Illich**

Patients may recover in spite of drugs or because of them. **– JH Gaddum**

The best physician is one who knows the worthlessness of the most medicines.
– Benjamin Franklin

Physiology is the step child of medicine. That is why Cinderella often turns out the queen.
– Martin H Fischer

Man is a creature composed of countless millions of cells: A microbe is composed of only one, yet throughout the ages the two have been in ceaseless conflict.
– AB Christie

Our profession is the only one which works unceasingly to annihilate itself.
– Martin H Fischer

The doctor may also learn more about the illness from the way the patient tells the story than from the story itself. **– James B Herrick**

Don't think of organ donations as giving up part of yourself to keep a total stranger alive. It's really a total stranger giving up almost all of themselves to keep part of you alive. **– Author Unknown**

Most of those evils we poor mortals know from doctors and imagination flow. **– Charles Churchill**

Men are not going to embrace eugenics. They are going to embrace the first likely, trimfigured. Don't take your organs to heaven with you. Heaven knows we need them here. **– Author Unknown**

For the most part, Western medicine doctors are not healers, preventers, listeners, or educators. But they're damned good at saving a life and the other aspects kick the beam. It's about time we brought some balance back to the scale. **– Claire Todae**

A sweating ovary or a sick prostate explains most history.
– Martin H Fischer

The only weapon with which the unconscious patient can immediately retaliate upon the incompetent surgeon is hemorrhage.
– William Stewart Halsted

The public blabbers about preventative medicine, but will neither appreciate nor pay for it. You get paid for what you cure. **– Martin H Fischer**

To save a man's life against his will is the same as killing him. **– Horace**

Nowadays the clinical history too often weighs more than the man.
– Martin H Fischer

Hypochondriacs squander large sums of time in search of nostrums by which they vainly hope they may get more time to squander.
– Mortimer Collins

One doctor makes work for another. **– English Proverb**

Doctors are just the same as lawyers; the only difference is that lawyers merely rob you, whereas doctors rob you and kill you, too.
– Anton Chekhov, Ivanov

Let the young know they will never find a more interesting, more instructive book than the patient himself. **– Giorgio Baglivi**

Formerly, when religion was strong and science weak, men mistook magic for medicine; now, when science is strong and religion weak, men mistake medicine for magic. **– Thomas Szasz**

My soul is dark with stormy riot, directly traceable to diet.
– Samuel Hoffenstein

The Lord hath created medicines out of the earth; and he that is wise will not abhor them. **– Ecclesiasticus**

Stomach: A slave that must accept everything that is given to it, but which avenges wrongs as slyly as does the slave. **– Emile Souvester**

A good digestion turneth all to health. **– George Herbert**

In Physic, things of melancholic hue and quality are used against melancholy, Sour against sour, salt to remove salt humours.
– John Milton

Our lives are not in the lap of the gods, but in the lap of our cooks.
– Lin Yutang

Opposites are cures for opposites. **– Hippocrates**

A man has often more trouble to digest food than to get it. **– Proverb**

Happiness for me is largely a matter of digestion. **– Lin Yutang**

A physician is obligated to consider more than a diseased organ, more even than the, whole man, he must view the man in his world.
– Harvey Cushing

Men of lean habit of body are commonly a long time healthy, having good appetites and strong stomachs for digestion. **– Tobias Venner**

Indigestion is charged by God with enforcing morality on the stomach.
– Victor Hugo

Ah me! love can not be cured by herbs. **– Ovid**

Foolish the doctor who despises the knowledge acquired by the ancients.
– Hippocrates

Life is not merely to be alive, but to be well. **– Marcus Valerius Martial**

The patient who takes medicine and neglects diet, wastes the skill of the physician. **– Chinese Proverb**

Let nothing which can be treated by diet be treated by other means.
– Maimonides

Even if conventional medicine tells you that your condition is incurable or that your only option is to live a life dependent on drugs with troublesome side effects, there is hope for improving or reversing your condition.
– Leon Chaitow

The treatments themselves do not 'cure' the condition, they simply restore the body's self-healing ability. **– Leon Chaitow**

Man is ill because he is never still. **– Paracelsus**

I believe that you can, by taking some simple and inexpensive measures, extend your life and your years of well-being. My most important recommendation is that you take vitamins everyday in optimun amounts, to supplement the vitamins you receive in your food. **– Linus Pauling**

Health is the proper relationship between microcosm, which is man, and the macrocosm, which is the universe. Disease is a disruption of this relationship. **– Dr Yeshe Donden, Physician to the Dalai Lama**

The art of medicine consists of amusing the patient while nature cures the disease. **– Voltaire**

The next major advance in the health of the American people will be determined by what the individual is willing to do for himself.
– John Knowles

Don't ask the doctor, ask the patient. **– Yiddish Proverb**

It may seem a strange principle to enunciate as the very first requirement in a hospital that it should do the sick no harm. **– Florence Nightingale**

A man may esteem himself happy when that which is his food is also his medicine. **– Henry David Thoreau**

Modern outlook has replaced to mean "Health" as a state of complete physical, mental and social well-being and not merely absence of disease or infirmity with an addition to include the ability to lead a socially and economically productive life.

Health Legislations

Some of the Constitutions in the world, which have come into existence after the Second World War, have specifically stated that right to health is a right which could be exercised against the State but in certain Constitutions such as ours, it is stated in an implied way.

The parliamentary laws such as Mental Health Act, Organ Transplantation Act, Sex Determination Act, Disabilities Act, Anti-pollution laws are some of the steps taken to regulate and improve the human activity to avoid any exploitation. Besides this, there are several other legislations in the field of health and public.

1947: Ministries of Health and Director-General of Health Services established at the Center and States. The Indian Nursing Council Act passed.

1948: India joined the World Health Organization (WHO) and the Employees State Insurance Act passed. The Dental Council of India established under the Dentist Act.

1949: The Registrar-General of India appointed in the Ministry of Home Affairs. The WHO opened its Southeast Asia Regional Office in New Delhi. The Indian Pharmacy Council and Family Planning Association of India established.

1950: India became a Republic in the Commonwealth. The Planning Commission was set up by the Government of India.

1951: The beginning of the First Five Year Plan. The BCG vaccination program launched in the country.

1952: The Community Development Program launched for the all-round rural development. The Central Council of Health constituted. First primary health center set up.

1953: The National Malaria Control Programme and National Extension Service Program for rural development started. A nationwide family planning programme started. A committee appointed to draft a Model Public Health Act for the country.

1954: The Contributory Health Service Scheme (Central Government Health Scheme), the Central Social Welfare Board, the National Water Supply and Sanitation Programme and the National Leprosy Control Programme started. The Prevention of Food Adulteration Act passed by the Parliament.

1955: The National Filaria Control Programme commenced. The National TB sample survey conducted.

1956: The Second Five-Year Plan started. The Model Public Health Act published and the Central Health Education Bureau established in the Union Health Ministry. The Indian Medical Council established.

1957: Influenza pandemic swept the country. The Demographic Research Centers established in Kolkata, Delhi and Trivandrum.

1958: The National Malaria Control Programme converted into National Malaria Eradication Programme. The National Development Council endorses Panchayati Raj. The National TB survey completed.

1959: The Mudaliar Committee appointed. A Central Expert Committee recommended eradication of small pox and cholera. Rajasthan introduces Panchayati Raj. National Tuberculosis Institute at Bangalore established.

1960: The School Health Committee and the National Nutrition Advisory Committee constituted.

1961: The Third Five-Year Plan launched. The Mudaliar Committee report published. The Central Bureau of Health Intelligence established.

1962: The Central Family Planning Institute established in Delhi. The National Smallpox eradication Programme and the School Health Programme initiated, the National Goitre Control Programme and the District Tuberculosis Programme launched.

1963: The Applied Nutrition Programme was launched with aid from the UNICEF, FAO and WHO. The National Institute of Communicable Diseases (formerly Malaria Institute of India) inaugurated and the National Trachoma Control Programme started. A Drinking Water Board and the Chadha Committee established.

1964: The National Institute of Health Administration and Education established.

1965: Reinforced Extended Family Planning Programme launched. The Mukherjee Committee set up.

1966: A separate department of Family Planning created under the Health Ministry. The Population Council's International Postpartum Family Planning Programme started in Delhi and Trivandrum.

1967: The Central Council of Health recommended levy of health cess on patients. The Jungalwala Committee set up.

1968: The Small Family Committee's Report submitted. Government appointed the Medical Education Committee.

1969: The Fourth Five-Year Plan launched. The Nutrition Research Laboratories became the National Institute of Nutrition. The Central Births and Deaths Registration Act promulgated.

1970: The Drugs (Price Control) Order promulgated. All India Hospital (Postpartum) Family Planning Programme started. The Population Council of India and the Central Council of Indian Medicine (Ayurveda, Unani and Siddha) formed. Voluntary Health Association of India (VHAI) comes into being.

1971: The Family Pension Scheme (FPS) for industrial workers came into force. The Medical Termination of Pregnancy Bill passed by the Parliament. Uni-purpose Health Workers converted into multipurpose workers.

1972: National Service Bill passed. The National Nutrition Monitoring Bureau set up.

1973: National Programme of Minimum Needs was incorporated in the Fifth Five-Year Plan. The Government envisaged a scheme for setting up 30-bedded rural hospitals; one such hospital for every 4 primary health centers. The Kartar Singh Committee recommended a new cadre of health workers called "Multipurpose Health Workers". The Central Council of Homeopathy set up.

1974: The Fifth Five-Year Plan launched. Parliament enacted the Water (Prevention and Control of Pollution) Act.

1975: India became smallpox-free. A Revised strategy for NMEP accepted. The "Integrated Child Development" scheme launched. The National Children's Welfare Board set up. The Cigarettes Regulation (Production, Supply and Distribution) Act passed by the Parliament. The Srivastava Committee set up.

1976: The Equal Remuneration Act promulgated providing for equal wages for men and women for equal work. A new Population Policy introduced. A National Programme for Prevention of Blindness formulated. The Central Council for Yoga and Naturopathy established.

1977: The National Institute of Health and Family Planning formed. The Rural Health Scheme launched. Community Health Volunteers (Guides) scheme taken up. "Population Control and Family Planning" was put in the concurrent list. The WHO adopted the goal of `Health for All by 2000 AD'.

1978: A Bill on Air Pollution introduced in the Lok Sabha. The Parliament approved the Child Marriage Restraint (Amendment Bill fixing the minimum age of marriage of 21 years for boys and 18 years for girls).

1979: The World Health Assembly endorsed the Declaration of 'Alma Ata' on primary health care.

1980: Smallpox officially declared eradicated from the entire world by the World Health Assembly. The Sixth Five-Year Plan launched.

1981: The census taken. The WHO and the member countries adopted the global strategy for 'Health for All.' The Report of the Working Group on Health for All, set up by the Planning Commission published. The first AIDS case detected in the country.

1982: The Government of India announced the National Health Policy. Amendment done on the Drugs and Cosmetics Act of 1940.

1984: The Bhopal Gas tragedy, the worst ever industrial accident killing at least 2500 people and no fewer than 50,000 affected. The ESI (Amendment) Bill approved by the Parliament and the Workmen's Compensation (Amendment) Act came into force.

1985: The Seventh Five-year Plan launched. The Universal Immunization Programme started. The Lepers Act, 1898, was repealed by the Parliament. A separate Department of Women and Child development set up under the newly created Ministry of Human Resource Development.

1986: The Environment (Protection) Act and the Consumer Protection Act were promulgated. National Drug Policy announced.

1987: The New 20-Point Programme launched. A worldwide "safe motherhood" campaign was launched by the World Bank. National Diabete Control Programme and National AIDS Control Programme initiated. Mental Health Act passed. The Drugs (Price Control) Order released.

1988: Hospitals and Other Institutions (Redressal of Grievances of Employees) Bill passed.

1989: Blood Safety Programme was launched. The ESI (Amendment) Act modified.

1990: Control of Acute Respiratory Infection (ARI) Programme initiated as a pilot project in 14 districts.

1991: India stages the last decadal Census of the century. Population of India was 844.32 million. Prenatal Diagnostic Techniques (regulation and prevention of misuse) Act enacted.

1992: Eighth Five-Year Plan launched. Child Survival and Safe Motherhood Programme (CSSM) launched in the country. The Infant Milk Substitute, Feeding Bottles and Infant Foods (Regulation of Production,

Supply and Distribution) Act passed. The State of India's Health Report by VHAI released.

1993: A major earthquake kills over 2000 people in Maharashtra.

1994: Return of Plague after 28 years of silence in few parts of the country. The Transplantation of Human Organs Bill passed. The first heart transplantation surgery in the country done at AIIMS, New Delhi. Malaria epidemic strikes Rajasthan. The Swaminathan Committee Report submitted.

1995: The revised Rational Drug Policy announced. Malaria epidemic strikes in Assam. The Persons with Disabilities (Equal Opportunities, Protection of Rights and Full Participation) Act passed.

1996: Dengue epidemic in Delhi. Malaria strikes again many in northern states of India. The Central Government publishes the 'list of essential drugs'. The Revised National TB Control Programme initiated. The Supreme Court orders the government to set up the National Council of Blood Transfusion.

1997: The National Illness Assistance Fund launched. Delhi government enacts Anti-smoking Bill. Subsequently, Anti-smoking Act at public places has been passed.

1998: National Institute of Pharmaceutical Education and Research Act.

1999: National Trust for Welfare of Persons with Autism, Cerebral Palsy, Mental Retardation and Multiple Disabilities Act.

2006: The Food Safety and Standards Act.

2008: The said legislation has been given effect recently to cover the public places.

Index

N

O

P

Q

R

S

T

U

V

W